THE
MODELING
HANDBOOK

The Complete Guide to Breaking into Local, Regional, and International Modeling

Third Edition

EVE MATHESON

An Owl Book

Henry Holt and Company
New York

Henry Holt and Company, Inc.
Publishers since 1866
115 West 18th Street
New York, New York 10011

Henry Holt® is a registered trademark
of Henry Holt and Company, Inc.

Published in Canada by Fitzhenry & Whiteside Ltd.,
195 Allstate Parkway, Markham, Ontario L3R 4T8.

Library of Congress Cataloging-in-Publication Data
Matheson, Eve.
The modeling handbook: the complete guide to breaking into local,
regional, and international modeling / Eve Matheson.—Rev. ed.
    p.   cm.
"An Owl book"
1. Models, Fashion—Vocational guidance—Handbooks, manuals,
etc.   2. Models, Fashion—Vocational guidance—United States—
Handbooks, manuals, etc.   I. Title.
HD6073.M77M38   1992
659.1'52—dc20   91-34884
                                                          CIP

ISBN 0-8050-3830-2 (An Owl Book: pbk.)

Henry Holt books are available for
special promotions and premiums.
For details contact: Director, Special Markets.

First published as *The World of International Modeling* in 1987.
First Owl Book Edition—1989
Third Edition—1995

Designed by Susan Hood
Printed in the United States of America
10 9 8 7 6 5 4 3 2 1

Dedicated with love to Solveig, Tracy—and Ian, a model husband.

Contents

Contents

A Note of Thanks

My sincere thanks to all of the model agents who took time out of very busy schedules to answer questions and supply information. Without their encouragement and support I could not have written this book. In addition to the many people interviewed I extend special thanks to Mr. Don Wightman and Miss Patt Vida. A very special bouquet to model agency receptionists and bookers all over the world, for their coffee, tea, and graciousness.

Introduction

This book is the result of extensive research, thousands of miles of travel around the world by plane, boat, hydrofoil, helicopter, bus, train, subway, bike, and foot (oh, the feet!), plus hundreds of interviews with models (male and female), agents, photographers, hairdressers, makeup artists, clients, casting directors, school directors, parents, and apartment owners. With my teenage daughter, Tracy, who has modeled in New York, Hamburg, Paris, and Milan, I went to the fashion capitals. Having spent a year in Europe, Tracy knew the problems of young men and women starting out in the modeling profession. Her experience and input were invaluable. We covered all the territory, asked question after question, experienced the problems, and found solutions.

My aim in writing this book is not to inflate or shatter dreams, but to help the thousands of young people who choose modeling as a career. Parents too will find the book invaluable in allowing them to learn about the business and its requirements.

ONE

1

Modeling—Is It for You?

Before we discuss in detail how to break into the modeling profession and pursue a successful career, it is important you know and understand some of the cold, hard facts of the profession.

Modeling is a multimillion-dollar, worldwide, closely knit business. Its growth in recent years has been phenomenal. Now it is show business, with thousands clamoring to get into the act. It is riddled with rejection, disillusionment, insecurity, depression, and frustration. Gossip travels like wildfire. Rumors fly around the world and ricochet back as fact. Reputations are ruined with a telephone call. Pressure rains down on everyone—client, agent, booker, photographer, and model. Competition dominates every phase of the industry. Despite crippling odds, a few make it to the top and become superstars. Others make large amounts of money but their names are never known. (Anonymity is a slim price to pay for a fat bank account and peace of mind.) The majority are devastated by disappointments and shattered dreams. At the start, it all seems so easy and glamorous. It is not. It is the cruelest profession of all!

It sounds shocking, doesn't it? But on the flip side, modeling is glamorous, fun, exciting, and extremely lucrative; it affords incredible opportunities for travel to the most exotic corners of the globe. Most successful models are happy and in control of their lives. They wouldn't change places with anyone. They make a lot of money and invest in the future, knowing that a model's career span is short. How did they realize their dream? What makes the difference between failure and success? There are many answers to these questions and you will find them all in this book. I am convinced that lack of knowledge of the modeling business and false information are two of the main reasons careers fail. The majority of young people have no idea what is involved in a modeling career or what it takes to get started and succeed. If you seriously want to be a professional model, study the following information and answer the questions honestly.

Over 100,000 young men and women will try to break into the modeling profession this year. Can you handle this kind of competition? Modeling means endless hours of hard work. Do you have the stamina? It means rejection on a daily basis. Can your ego stand it? The first three months must be considered a financial investment on your part as well as your agent's. Do you have at least a thousand dollars in the bank? An easy smile, happy disposition, neat appearance, inner sparkle, and professional attitude are essential. Do you have these attributes? It can take months to launch a fledgling model's career. Is patience one of your virtues? Fashion models must be at least 5'9" tall and fit a size six to eight. Are you slim enough and tall enough—without heels? Good bone structure, perfect teeth, and beautiful skin are also essential. Do you have all of these? If you are too short for fashion, are you prepared to find a commercial agent and take acting lessons and television and photo-posing workshops to prepare you for the camera? Modeling is very stressful, especially for the beginner who has to deal with bookers, clients, photographers, stylists, makeup artists, designers, and fashion editors as well as having to run all over town and be punctual for all appointments. Can you handle the stress? Lack of confidence is your greatest foe. Can you believe in yourself enough to overcome it? Being pretty doesn't necessarily mean you are photogenic. Do you photograph well? Are you healthy? Are you emotionally stable? Can you say no to drugs? *(You must!)* Do you have great energy? Above all, do you have a burning desire to be a model and absolute determination to succeed? If the answer to all of these questions is a resounding yes, then modeling *is* for you.

2

How to Get Started

"I want to be a model. How can I get started?" I hear these words regularly from young men and women all over the country. There are a number of approaches. A lot depends on your age, height, and where you live.

First let's talk about girls. If you are sixteen or seventeen years old and 5'9" tall, weigh 120 pounds, have good cheekbones, a beautiful complexion, and long legs, you have an excellent chance of being accepted by a top agent in a major market. Have a couple of snapshots or Polaroids taken by a friend or relative. One of these should be a head shot showing your face and hair, the other a body shot showing your legs. If you have a bathing-suit picture you can use that too. I emphasize that you do not need to spend hundreds of dollars to have pictures taken by a professional photographer. The top model agents don't like posed pictures or portraits. They want to see you looking relaxed and natural. If you live in or near a major market such as New York, Chicago, Dallas, or Los Angeles, telephone the major agencies (I have listed them in the chapters discussing those markets, or you can find them in the classified pages of the telephone directory) and ask if they have open calls, a time set aside each week to see new faces. Take your pictures in at the appointed time. If you are trying your luck with several agencies you will obviously need several copies. Be sure to put your name, address, and telephone number on the back of each photograph. A trained agent will know within seconds if you have potential, and the decision to accept you will be made rapidly. If there are too many girls at the open calls to be seen individually, you will be asked to leave the photographs and you will be contacted later.

If you don't live near a major market, mail your pictures to the agencies and include a stamped, self-addressed envelope and a letter requesting an interview, the return of your pictures, and the agent's comments. Generally you will receive a reply along the lines of: "We'd love to see you. . . ." or "You are not our type. . . ." When an interview is granted you will have to pay any travel or hotel expenses you incur.

Perhaps you fulfill the ideal model's requirements but don't feel confident or mature enough to live and work in a major market, or you are under 5'9" and therefore could not work in such an area at this stage. The best plan here is to start out at a regional or local level. Seattle, San Francisco, Atlanta, and Miami are good regional markets. Follow exactly the same procedure for the open calls or send a letter requesting an interview.

On the local level, check your telephone book for model agencies and call to ask if you might send pictures. If they agree, send them off and follow up with a telephone call a few days later. If you are concerned about the reputation of an agency check it out with the Better Business Bureau, the chamber of commerce, or the industrial commission of the state in which you live. You can also check credentials with the closest offices of the Screen Actors Guild (SAG) or the American Federation of Television and Radio Artists (AFTRA). These are the two main unions for actors and models. You might have to write or call the head offices for the nearest branch: Screen Actors Guild, 5757 Wilshire Blvd., Los Angeles, CA 90036, Tel. (213) 954-1600; AFTRA, 260 Madison Avenue—7th Floor, New York, NY 10016, Tel. (212) 532-0800.

Be wary of MODELS WANTED advertisements in your local paper. And *never* arrange to meet or go anywhere with an agent, scout, or photographer who stops you in the street. Accept his or her business card and investigate thoroughly.

If you do not have a model agency in your area I suggest you call on the fashion buyers of your local department stores, or owners of boutiques, and ask if you might model in upcoming fashion shows. Write to the fashion editor of your local newspaper or magazine and offer to model for a fashion feature. Call on reputable photographers in your area and ask if they could use you for commercial work.

Another category of would-be model is the thirteen- to fifteen-year-old who has to finish school. This is an excellent time to lay the groundwork for an exciting future. If you are really interested in becoming a model, read as many magazines as possible and learn about the modeling profession. To gain confidence take part in school, church, or local fashion shows. A teen modeling or self-improvement course at a department store would be a wise investment. Videos explaining runway techniques or special makeup skills for on-camera work are also good investments. If you have a weight problem, now is the time to overcome it permanently by developing good eating habits and exercising regularly. Stay away from drugs and alcohol. If you develop a dependency on any of these, modeling is out of the question. Smoking is also a health hazard.

The prospective male model should know that he is in a female-dominated profession. There is no equality of the sexes in pay or job opportunities. The big consolation is that a man's career lasts much longer. He can work from the age of nineteen to forty-five or over. Height requirements for men are 6′0″ to 6′2″, jacket size 40 Regular or Long, waist 31–32, sleeve 33–35, neck 15½–16½.

The game plan for getting started is the same as for girls. You should send snapshots and a letter to the all-male agencies or agencies with divisions for men. I have listed these in the various cities. Be assured that Americans are the most popular male models in the world.

We have explored the different age levels and categories and the direct approach to starting a career. Here are some other approaches worth consideration.

Competitions and Model Searches

Beware of scams! If you are suspicious of an event, call the Better Business Bureau and investigate. If, however, these events are legitimate, they can open up excellent career opportunities, as a couple of success stories will illustrate: Kristin Salo, a six-foot-tall beauty and a 4.0 honor student from Lutz, Florida, won the runway division of the Talent Search of America event in Tampa, Florida. The end result was a meeting with Eileen Ford, owner of Ford Models Inc. in New York, and a modeling contract.

Super model Beverly Peele was twelve years old and 5′9″ when she won a local modeling contest in California, her home state. The prize was a scholarship to a modeling school. The school entered her in another contest, where Beverly won prize money and an opportunity to attend the International Model and Talent Association Convention in Los Angeles. Beverly was an immediate success; she was signed by a Los Angeles agency and worked in New York and Milan where she modeled the Collections. A year later she appeared on the cover of *Mademoiselle*. What a way to start a career!

Modeling Conventions

The International Model and Talent Association Convention is an outstanding event held in Los Angeles in January and in New York in July. It offers unparalleled opportunities for launching a career in the modeling or acting professions. Participants are seen by top casting directors and some of the most prestigious agents in the world.

There are many conventions held all over this country and Canada. It is important that you investigate them thoroughly before you invest any money. The chapter on competitions and conventions will help you evaluate these events.

Modeling School Courses

A modeling school course is not essential to a career in modeling. It can be of great value, however, if it is run by experienced professionals who are, or have been, associated with the modeling profession.

When you visit a school study the curriculum carefully. Make sure it covers essential aspects of your prospective career such as runway technique, hair and makeup instruction, wardrobe, photographic posing, television commercial workshops, acting classes, and in-depth discussions of the industry.

Here are some questions you should ask: Is the school licensed by the state department of education? Is it bonded? Does it have an agency and if so, is that agency bonded and licensed? If it does not have an agency, does it have an affiliation with one? What are its connections with the major agencies around the country? Is it involved with a modeling association of the caliber of the International Model and Talent Association? What are the school's graduates doing—have some of them gone on to successful modeling careers? What are the present students doing? Are they modeling in the best fashion shows in town? Are they working for the best advertising agencies and photographers?

Christiev Carothers was an international model before opening one of the most successful modeling schools in the country in Medford, Oregon. She is also a model scout which means she has firsthand knowledge of what it takes to make a model. She said: "I went to a modeling school course years ago and it changed my life forever. I learned so much. Unfortunately these courses always seem to have a scam stigma attached to them. The problems start when schools promise students they will be stars. Everyone who goes to school will encounter more and gain more. That's a guarantee. But very few will go on to be models—I won't even say stars."

Alecia Bell, of the International Top Models Agency in Toronto, Canada, told me: "There are a lot of scams that take advantage of young girls. I see girls who have spent a thousand dollars on a portfolio. They come to my agency and I can't take them because they are too short. I do work with a few fabulous schools that are very up-to-date, and their instructors are trained to the ultimate. If a school has a very up-to-date curriculum and good teachers—that's super. But super girls are often taught bad habits and outdated techniques, and it is a nightmare to have to retrain them."

Eileen Green, who owned and operated the Eileen Green Agency in Hamburg, Germany, for many years, told me: "A modeling school course is important for any young girl because she will learn deportment and self-confidence. Even if she never enters the modeling world, it is not money wasted. It can help her with any career. But I do think every school should have at least one lecture telling prospective models how to survive in Europe." In Paris, Nicolas Fiani, a partner in SAGA Models, said: "School directors in America must be strong enough to look at a girl who is 5'2" and weighs 150 pounds and tell her that she can't model in Paris."

Jack Rasnic, founder and coordinator of the Models of the South convention, said: "Modeling schools have become better educated in ascertaining skills that major agencies require of their models. Everyone has discovered that a professional model cannot be just a pretty face; she must have skills in photography and acting as well as runway.''

English-born Diane Whittacker-Muth of Florida has had over twenty years experience as a professional model and teacher. Among her many success stories is Gina Swainson who became Miss World, 1979. Diane told me: ''A good modeling school teaches young people responsibility, poise, confidence, the importance of being on time, professionalism of image, and how to accept rejection, as well as runway and makeup techniques. These are things that are not only important for the modeling field, but for all walks of life.''

The Agency Interview

This can make or break a career, so your attitude at the interview is very important. You must be pleasant, positive, and alert. Turn nervousness into energy. If the agent is having a twinge of doubt, a nice personality will weight the decision in your favor. Answer questions honestly and ask as many as you need; remember, the interview serves both parties. Shake hands at the beginning and at the end. Don't wear too much makeup, and avoid bizarre hairdos! Wear an outfit you have worn before and in which you feel comfortable: you must look and feel great. Stay away from silk, which can make you perspire, and likewise don't wear layers of clothing. Wear a dress, or skirt and blouse, that will show your figure and legs.

As you can see, there are many ways to get started in a modeling career, depending on your location, age, and type. Believe in yourself! Don't be afraid to try! And don't give up your dreams!

3

Explanation of Modeling Terms

To help you understand this book more clearly, here are some of the terms used in the modeling profession.

Book or Portfolio

This contains the photographs and tear sheets that show a client examples of your work.

Tear Sheets

These are pages from magazines and other publications that show a model at work. Since tear sheets indicate experience they are essential credentials.

Testing

Testing is the term used for a photographic session to produce pictures for your portfolio and composite.

Go-Sees

A go-see is a job interview with a photographer or a client.

Casting

A casting is an interview for a television commercial.

Callback

This is a second audition for a job.

Option

This is the term used when a model's assignment is put on hold because weather conditions are questionable or because the final decision to book him or her has not yet been made.

Dresser

This is the person who will help you change into various outfits with lightning speed backstage at a fashion show. Don't scream, slap, or swear at the dresser! You couldn't do the job without her.

Head Shot

A close-up photograph of a model's head and face.

Headsheet

An agency will usually have a book containing pictures and statistics of all of their models and/or a headsheet, which is a large sheet of paper containing the same details. This information is mailed to clients and is very instrumental in obtaining work. You will have to pay to be included in headsheets.

A Shoot

Time spent in a studio or on location with a photographer or camera crew for an assignment.

On Location

This is where the shoot takes place. It can be a place you know well or an exotic spot on the other side of the world. This is your opportunity to travel, with all expenses paid including your salary.

Voucher

A voucher is a payment form and a contract between you and the client. It is essential that you fill these out correctly. The procedure is that you give a copy to the client, retain a copy, and give a third copy to your agency immediately so that billing can be done without delay. (Never allow a photographer or client to add any conditions to the voucher or delete any reference to reproduction rights. And never sign a paper relinquishing reproduction rights without the approval of your agency.)

Composite, Card, Index Card (in England), or Sed Card

The above terms all mean the same. The Sed Card is named after its inventor, Sebastian Sed of the former Parker-Sed Agency in Germany. It is a group of pictures on one card showing a model in different poses and with different expressions. The card lists height, weight, and measurements, and the name and telephone number of the model's agency. It is a very important tool and should only be put together with the help of a legitimate, knowledgeable, and experienced agent.

Mother Agent

The mother agent is the name given to the agent who handles the model and successfully introduces him or her to the international scene.

Terms Describing the Main Types of Modeling

Live Modeling

This refers to runway, showroom, fitting, and trade-show work. Runway models are fashion models who work at local, regional and international levels. The most exciting runway work is done at the haute couture (high fashion) designer shows in New York, Paris, Milan, and London. Models must be at least 5′9″ tall and have a 34″ hip measurement and great stamina. In showrooms, models wear manufacturers' clothing for buyers of department and chain stores. A trade-show model will represent a client's product at a trade show.

Photographic Modeling

This has two categories. The first is editorial, or print, which is excellent for prestige, your portfolio, and your ego! The pay is not very good, however, with the day rate ranging from $120 to $250 for a magazine cover. The big payoff comes from the exposure, which attracts advertising or commercial clients.

Television Commercials

This is an extremely well paid category in this country, but not in Europe. In the United States it has made modeling the multimillion-dollar industry it is today.

Catalog Modeling

As the name implies, this is for the production of catalogs. It is steady work and pays well. Hamburg, Germany; Melbourne, Australia; Miami, Chicago, and Dallas are very big markets. Movie star Nick Nolte started out as a catalog model.

4

Problems and Solutions

What are the major problems associated with the modeling profession? Who is to blame for the hundreds of disappointed young men and women in New York and the fashion capitals of Europe? Why did their dreams turn into nightmares?

I talked to models at every level of success. I found there were far too many of them at the bottom of the ladder without a hope of making it to the first rung. They had been misinformed about the industry and told that modeling in Europe would be easy. They had been told that within three months they would have enough tear sheets and experience to return to New York and make a lot of money. It hadn't taken long for them to realize that they had been misled. Having arrived with insufficient funds to support themselves, they had no money left and no means of getting home.

Blame is an unpleasant word. So let us use *responsibility*. Responsibility lies heavily on those who give technicolor impressions of future success without actually making concrete promises. Many self-styled experts have never been to Europe. They have no idea what international modeling involves.

Responsibility also lies heavily with parents. Many push their children into modeling careers. The pressure experienced by young models in Europe from parents—especially mothers—is appalling! Young people themselves must also share the responsibility. My advice to them is to be sensible and face the facts. If you are not the right height, shape, or don't have the correct personality, and if an agent has discouraged you from going into the business, take the advice and ignore the urgings of an anxious mother or a school director. If you are fortunate enough to be signed by an agent, enjoy one starry-eyed moment and then get down to business. Ask questions and learn about your profession.

For the young model overseas, here are the problems and suggested solutions:

Homesickness

Homesickness is the first problem, but it is quickly overcome. You will be so busy moving into your new home, meeting clients and photographers, and posing for test sessions, that at the end of the day you will be too tired to think of being homesick. The answer is to throw yourself into your new career and make friends with other new models as quickly as possible. You can have a great time exploring the city and taking side trips on weekends.

Culture Shock

In the beginning, this is the biggest and most serious problem. A model must adapt to new customs, fashions, food, lifestyles, languages, currencies, and transportation—and all at the same time. One is forced to adapt quickly. Worrying about these changes will affect your looks, attitude, and performance. A good solution is to read as much as possible in advance about the country where you will be working. You can also rent a video, which is an exciting way to see and learn.

Another solution is to spend time with a foreign-exchange teller at a bank in order to learn the currency of the country. Find German, French, and Italian groups in your hometown and ask them to tell you about their country and its customs. (People are always pleased to brag about their country.) Study foreign-language magazines. When you arrive in Europe talk to models—especially those from your own country—and listen to their explanations of why life is different. Talk to your booker and agent. They are always delighted when models show an interest in something other than modeling. And above all, *don't criticize local people and customs*—at least not in public. Their ways may not be yours, but that does not make them wrong. My daughter Tracy was most indignant when an old lady on the subway in Hamburg rapped her on the knee and told her to uncross her legs. Tracy's companion, who was also a model, received withering looks because she was wearing a short skirt. A girl who crosses her legs or wears short skirts is frowned upon by the older generation in Germany.

American friendliness, which as a foreigner I find charming, is sometimes misunderstood in Europe. Europeans are more reserved (with the possible exception of people in ski lines!). The delightful American eagerness to make friends is often misinterpreted as pushiness. You must be polite, courteous, and quiet in restaurants and public places. You will be accepted graciously if you try to blend into that society and respect the customs. Good manners are important no matter what nationality you are or what country you are in.

Learning to deal with culture shock is an education. You will become more confident and independent. Within the first month, you will have broadened your outlook and expanded your knowledge.

Language Barriers

It is overwhelming to arrive in a country and not know a word of the language. You cannot make a telephone call or order a meal. Radio and television sound like gibberish, and by the end of the day you are totally exhausted, not just from climbing thousands of stairs (elevators are unheard of in the older buildings in Europe) but from being constantly surrounded by foreign words and sounds.

Trying to find your way around town can be most distressing. Let me give you an example of my personal experience. When I was in Hamburg, my daughter Tracy wanted me to understand how difficult and frightening it is for a young model to find her way to assignments in a foreign city where she does not understand the language or the transportation system and cannot afford the luxury of taxis. To enable me to appreciate all of this, Tracy set up six hypothetical go-sees in various parts of Hamburg. She established a time limit and insisted I use only bus or subway transportation. I pleaded with her to accompany me but she refused, explaining (smugly) that as she knew how to get to these destinations it would defeat the object of the exercise if she came. I was haunted by her final words: "I will *know* if you cheat and take a taxi!" It was a frightening experience. I did not do well, to say the least. Within fifteen minutes, I had broken the law. I had leaped onto a train (which was going in the wrong direction) without a ticket, and I was lost! The next few hours were a nightmare. I arrived (late) for two of the fictitious go-sees, bungled all other attempts to reach other destinations, and arrived back at the hotel (by taxi!) in a crumpled heap. A gleeful Tracy opened the taxi door with a loud "Tsk-Tsk!" and "Now, wasn't that easy? I can't wait until we get to Milan—you don't speak Italian either!"

One solution is to buy a beginner's foreign-language tape for your destination country. Play it constantly. Listen to it while you fall asleep and when you are on the plane. You

21

will be amazed at how many phrases you will pick up. Your ear will become accustomed to the sounds. A phrase book comes with each cassette. Keep it with you. Learn a few words each day. This will be a great help.

Tear Sheets

First of all, avoid the misconception that in Europe it is easy to get tear sheets and make money quickly. This is quite wrong. It is an established fact that tear sheets are an essential tool if a model is to work in New York. These days it is also an established fact that European clients are insisting more and more on booking experienced models who already have tear sheets. Consequently, it has become increasingly hard for a new model to work. In many cases, European tear sheets are needed in order to work in Europe. It is a vicious cycle.

It is also discouraging to discover that a tear sheet that brings you work in Switzerland will be taken out of your book in Milan because it is unsuitable for that market. So when you are told, in essence, that Europe is that "big tear sheet in the sky," don't believe it. Know that it will take time and money to get tear sheets that are good enough for your portfolio. Be prepared for this and be patient. Don't get discouraged—they will come eventually. Another point, however, is that even when you have done a job that will produce tear sheets, it will be some time before these are available to you. Fashion magazines are shot months ahead of publication, and by the time they are on the market you may well have moved on to another country. Ask your booker, another model, or a friend to keep an eye out for them and send them to you. It is frustrating to have worked and to have nothing to show for it. Clients are not interested in explanations; they want to see evidence of work.

Money

Some models starve and live in appalling conditions because they don't have enough money. Many fall prey to bad situations because they don't have enough money. How much money is enough? Apart from Japan, where the business is run quite differently (I have explained all of this in the chapter on Tokyo), a model should have sufficient funds to support him or herself for the first three months. An American, for instance, should take at least $1,500 to $2,000 to Europe plus a return ticket or additional funds for it. Insufficient money is a big problem and leads to other problems. But I warn you, *do not travel with cash*. Use travelers checks and, if possible, have at least one credit card. (A young photographer who arrived in Milan had his passport stolen en route and $2,400 in cash stolen within hours of his arrival in the city. He had to return to the United States.)

Why do you need this amount of money? First of all, it will take two or three weeks, probably even longer, to put together a composite or have pictures taken that are good enough to take on go-sees. (At this point, do not rush out for a session with a hometown photographer who doesn't know the European market. The photographer will make money and you will be left with useless prints.) A good idea is to find some current foreign magazines that will show you what "look" is in, in the various fashion capitals. A few photographs of this type would be a help to you and your European agent. Remember, a couple of good pictures are worth a dozen mediocre ones. (And unfortunately the bad ones are always remembered!) You will need money for food, for rent (even if an agent advances money, it has to be paid back— nothing is free!), for transportation, and for many incidentals.

Unprofessional Behavior

Throughout this book agents, successful models, and photographers stress the importance of professional behavior. What exactly does this mean? First, let me give you an example of unprofessional behavior and its consequences. A young English model on a rapid rise to fame in Europe became conceited, overconfident, and careless. She knew she was much in demand and thought clients and her agent would tolerate her less than professional attitude. She arrived late for work on several occasions. One day she didn't show up at all. A furious client called her agent, who in turn called the model's apartment. A boyfriend answered and told the agent that the girl had been working so much(!) she was tired and had decided not to go to work. The agent told the boyfriend to tell the girlfriend to come to the agency to pick up all her belongings. By the time the stunned model arrived her magazine covers, which had adorned the walls, had already been replaced by another beautiful face. No amount of tears would change the agent's mind. The agency's reputation was on the line. The model was finished.

Professional behavior means being reliable, punctual, adaptable, considerate, pleasant, and loyal to your agent. And here are a few other pointers for fledgling models. A go-see is not an opportunity for a gossip session with other models while you are waiting to see a client. This time should be spent concentrating on what you are going to say and do when your turn comes. Don't ask to see another model's portfolio and don't show yours to anyone but the client. Your book is *your* business.

When you meet the client, smile, shake hands, introduce yourself, and give the name of your agency. If you are nervous, transform your jitters into energy and enthusiasm. *Don't ever apologize for a weak portfolio!* If it isn't as good as it might be, spark the client's interest with your attitude and personality. Learn from successful models. Superstar Carol Alt attributes much of her phenomenal success to her professionalism. She told me: "There are many girls out there far better looking than I but you will never find one who is more professional." Follow Carol's advice. Be professional. Eliminate unprofessional behavior before it becomes a habit that will ruin your career.

Coping with the Unexpected

Sometimes actions speak louder than words. I was at a fashion show recently when a model lost one of her shoes on the runway. She reached down, took off the other shoe, and continued, without missing a beat. Remember this tip, if this should ever happen to you!

Airline Tickets

Take the time to shop around for your overseas airline ticket. Your agent will advance money for your fare, but if you can pay for it yourself it is better. You will eventually have to reimburse your agent; therefore, the cheaper the ticket the better off you will be. A word of warning, however. Make sure the airline is reputable and not likely to go out of business while you are in Europe. You could be left with a useless return ticket. Leave the return date open.

Here is another important point. Some large cities have more than one airport, so make sure connecting flights are from the same airport. Making a frantic dash from one airport to another is expensive and takes a lot of time.

I speak from experience. The day my daughter and I left for Europe I discovered that the airline we had planned to use had gone out of business. I had been in China until three days before our departure and had not heard of the airline's problems. Fast work by a travel agent secured two seats on a flight to London's Heathrow Airport. On the plane, I realized that our Paris flight departed from Gatwick. It would

25

have been impossible to make the connection on time had my family not met us at Heathrow and rushed us through the terminal to a helicopter, which took us to Gatwick. We arrived in the nick of time, made the connection, and met the agency representative in Paris as planned. It was a nerve-racking experience. It would have created a major problem for a young model and a distressing start to a career. So make sure you are booked on a reputable airline and that your flights arrive and leave from the same airport.

Overweight

Being overweight is not just another problem; it is a disaster! Don't go overseas hoping to lose a few extra pounds en route or within a few days of arrival. Lose weight before you go. You will be weighed and measured on the first day at your new agency. Believe me, they will not be happy if you are overweight. It will hold up your progress, because a reputable agent will not lie about your weight on a composite. In Europe, they talk in centimeters. There are 2.54 of these little horrors to every inch. A few centimeters too many will mean that you won't work in fashion or catalog. As every agent told me, the bottom line is that models have to fit into the clothes! And a new model must have as much of the market available as possible.

To help avoid this overweight problem, here are some tips on weight control. Foods are made up of: a) carbohydrates (2.4 calories per gram), b) proteins (2.4 calories per gram), and c) fats (4.8 calories per gram). Fats have twice the calories per gram and must therefore be watched and reduced in the diet. There are 3,500 calories in a pound of body weight. To control weight you must understand the intake and output of these calories. Well, we all know about intake! Output means exercise. You lose as many calories by walking as by running one mile; it just takes longer to walk. Your weight in pounds, multiplied by two-thirds, is the number of calories lost by running or walking a mile. To calculate the basic number of calories required to sustain your body weight when you are not exercising, multiply your present weight by 12 if you are a man (e.g. a 150-pound male requires 1,800 calories per day); and multiply by 11 if you are a woman (e.g. a 124-pound woman requires 1,364 calories per day). So, it is really quite easy to lose a pound a week, or even more, by reducing caloric intake and exercising. You will need an accurate list of calories contained in various foods. This can be obtained from a doctor, dietician, or reliable literature. Extra pounds mean tension, worry, depression, more eating, more weight gain, and so on. Don't let it happen to you!

Excess Luggage

Still on the problem of weight but a different kind, let's take a look at the problem of excess baggage. It is expensive to fly with luggage that is overweight, and it is also an unnecessary expense to have to store it. Also, it is a nuisance to have at your destination. Remember, hand luggage is not the excess that will not fit into your suitcase. I met one young model who had problems with both types of weight. She had paid $200 for excess baggage across the Atlantic, and a further $200 on a rowing machine, in a vain attempt to lose the weight she had gained since signing the contract with her agent. What a disaster!

Rejection and Depression

These two problems seem to go hand in hand. From the moment you become a model you must face the fact that no matter how pretty or handsome you are, or how perfect your measurements, you are going to be rejected over and over again by clients and photographers. It happens all the time—even to people at the top. It is part of the business. You must learn to live with it. It helps if you understand that the reason you do not get a particular job is not personal; it is because you are not the right type or the look for that particular job. It also helps if you know that you *will* work eventually. Be determined not to get depressed. I remember sitting in one agency in Paris, waiting for an interview, when a gorgeous model came back from a go-see and announced to the world—and her agent—''Well, they absolutely hated me there. What's next?'' With a brilliant smile, she took the details of her next go-see and breezed out. That model had the right attitude. She was positive. She was rolling with the punches.

Modeling is no place for the emotionally insecure. And don't forget: when the chips are down, you can always turn to the Super Agent. The power of prayer is amazing.

Insurance

The problem of accident and hospital costs can be avoided by having insurance before you leave home. *This is imperative!* In some countries, you will be covered by insurance after you have worked for a while. Find out the details of this from your foreign agent. To be on the safe side, take out health and accident insurance for the first three months.

Inadequate Business Knowledge

Insufficient knowledge of the modeling profession and the situation abroad can be a big problem. Far too many young men and women believe that because they have been accepted by a foreign agent, their dreams of becoming a successful international model are soon to be realized. This is a reasonable assumption, but it doesn't happen that easily. When a foreign agent agrees to take you overseas, it means that he or she believes that you have what it takes to model in that country, but there are no guarantees. That agent will work for you because that is the way he or she makes a living. This can take time.

Do not go overseas unless you have an agent at home who

understands the overseas business and will keep track of your progress. A good agent will know exactly how you should be treated and how your career should be handled. Make sure that your school director and your parents ask the questions that need to be answered. Parents must know exactly what their sons and daughters are getting into. They should know about accommodations, commissions, and finances. All agents have a list of rules and regulations concerning their agencies and policies. Ask for the details.

Excessive Drinking

Excessive drinking is a problem, especially in Germany, which is the first port of call for many new models and where the legal drinking age is fifteen. Wild parties and undisciplined behavior result in models being dropped by the agency and even sent home.

Drugs

To be caught with drugs means imprisonment and deportation. A model messing with drugs eventually loses everything. Agents will not tolerate the unreliability and substandard appearance that ensues.

MADA, which stands for Models Against Drug Abuse, was started by Tom and J. J. Meier of the Facefinders organization. MADA is one of a number of charities Facefinders supports in local communities during model searches at shopping malls around the country. Facefinders address: 3191 Tucker, Rossmore, CA 90720. Tel.(714) 828-FACE.

The Playboy Scene

A girl who is well balanced, has a strong sense of self-esteem, and has been well informed by her mother agent will not have a problem in this area. There are some very handsome men in Paris and Milan with gorgeous accents who like to surround themselves with beautiful girls. The parties, limousines, furs, and gifts are enticing, but the price is too high. When a stranger phones and invites you to a party, say no the first time and the second time and then you will probably be left alone. Modeling is a serious business. Late-night parties and drugs will affect your appearance and cost you your career, your self-respect, and possibly your life. Just say no. You don't need to do these things to be a successful model.

Stress

Stress is a model's enemy. It diminishes sparkle and self-esteem. I have seen many young people lose jobs because tension and pressure made them appear inexperienced or lacking in personality. Don't be a victim of stressful situations. Build your confidence. Listen to compliments and constructive comments from people who are guiding your career. You will soon learn to recognize what is genuine. Dwell on the good remarks. Think only positive thoughts. Always treat other people as you yourself would like to be treated. If a booker or agent is hostile give him or her the benefit of the doubt. They are probably stressed to the limit at that moment. Respond with kindness and understanding. A smile always helps. Next time around some of your pleasantness will probably have rubbed off on them.

Here are some exercises to help ward off tension. Try to do them twice a day even when you are *not* being stalked by doom. First, learn this breathing exercise: Take several long, slow, deep breaths, saying to yourself the word R-E-L-A-X. Think R-E while breathing in, and L-A-X while breathing out. Now, starting at the toes, work through the body, and work upwards, relaxing these muscle groups: Breathe in and out while tightening and loosening the toes, the calves, the thighs, and the buttocks. Exhale and relax. Breathe, and push your stomach out. Exhale and relax. Now do the chest, arms, shoulders, and neck area, crushing the arms to the ribs, tightening fists, and hunching shoulders as you inhale. Exhale and relax. Finally, breathe in as you close the eyes tightly, and tense the facial muscles. Exhale and relax. Take a few more deep breaths, remembering to repeat the word *relax*. . . . Now you are ready to pat yourself on the back and take on the world!

Finally, take heart. Even models at the peak of their careers have problems. One top model told me: "There is insecurity at the top. Most models have to worry about weight, and we are always looking over our shoulders to see who the next superstar will be. But the biggest problem is that we tend to become totally turned inward and to think only of ourselves. It is important to be interested in other people and subjects outside of modeling."

5

Legal Matters

This invaluable advice on a model's legal rights comes from Colin C. Claxon of San Rafael, California, an entertainment attorney whose practice includes representation of models and agencies. With his wife, Lynn, Colin co-owns the very successful Stars agency in San Francisco. His legal expertise and working knowledge of the modeling profession make him an authority on this subject. Here is what Colin has to say:

With all the glamour, glitter, excitement, energy, and world travel, modeling is, for everyone in it, a business. And everyone in it—the agent, booker, photographer, stylist, client, and *you*—is in it for the money, usually lots of it!

The business world is run on contracts, commitments, and definitions of what is expected, and the world of modeling is no exception. You must have a basic understanding of what you can expect and what is expected of you; a mistake may be costly—for you.

THE AGENCY CONTRACT

Most agencies require you to sign a contract, which is usually exclusive: you agree that you will not model or accept a booking except through that agency, and the agency agrees to locate bookings for you, and expects to receive a commission, usually 20 percent from you and a like amount from the client. While most contracts appear to prohibit you from working for other agencies or switching during the contract term (usually one [1] year), they are usually terminable by either party or by mutual agreement. Although contractual in nature, such contracts are essentially moral commitments.

If an agency treats its models as exclusive and you accept a booking from another agent or on your own, the agency can and will terminate you, and you have breached a valuable confidence and harmed your reputation in what is really a small community worldwide.

Often agency contracts include (in the contract itself, or in an additional document), rules or guidelines setting forth what the agency expects from you, agency policies, and specific procedures. These rules are binding on you. They may include such terms as repayment by you of expenses advanced by the agency for your development. Read and understand everything that you are given and ask questions until you have all the answers.

Agency contracts typically provide that the agency will bill the client for your services and receive the payment for you, and permit them to cash your check pursuant to a power of attorney contained in the contract, even if the check is in your name. They will deduct their commission and pay the balance to you. This is standard procedure. Most agencies pay at least every two (2) weeks if they have agreed to advance your payments. Some charge an additional 5 percent for that service. The alternative is to wait until the agency is paid, commonly 30–120 days after the booking. Your agency contract will usually provide that the agency can also deduct any monies advanced or loaned to you and all expenses paid on your behalf. Such expenses will include testing fees of photographers, film and print costs, long-distance phone calls you made from the agency or the model's apartment, Federal Express or other special delivery charges (domestic or international), forwarding your book to other agencies, rent and living expenses, and more. Be sure that you read your contract carefully for the right of the agency to deduct such costs with or without your advance approval. Never be afraid to ask in advance which charges you may be expected to pay, because the practice varies from agency to agency. Always demand an accounting and explanation for all such deductions.

The agency should not mark up or make a profit on such expenses; the deductions should represent the actual cost, nothing more. An exception is housing provided by agencies, who typically may charge private apartment rent for a facility shared with many other models, as a way of allocating the cost. Your mother agency should be able to negotiate a maximum that will be charged to you for such a shared arrangement.

If your agency places you with an agency in another city (or a foreign country), your original agent is the "mother" agency. The mother agency holds your contract and they are in charge of your career development. The two agencies will be sharing commissions on your bookings, but the total agency commissions you pay should not increase. While you are working elsewhere, you should stay in touch with the mother agency. Never permit another agency to alter your appearance, i.e., cut your hair, without discussing that with your mother agency. If you feel it is necessary to change agencies, do so only after consulting with your mother agency and obtaining their permission. Disagreements with the out-of-town agency should be referred to your mother agency. Taking care of you continues to be a part of their job.

THE VOUCHER

All agencies utilize some form of multipart voucher for each booking, for each model. Usually you will be given a book or package of blank vouchers. Be sure you read and understand each line and blank on the voucher form before you depart for your first booking. It is your responsibility to complete the voucher fully and correctly, and if the information given to you on the set or at the shoot varies from what you understood when you accepted the job, call your agent from the shoot before you leave and clarify any doubts. (In fact, if any problem occurs on the set insist on stopping and calling your agent before proceeding with the shoot; that is the time to solve the problem.) Never permit the client or photographer to alter the voucher in any way. Be sure that you obtain a signature on the voucher and that you return the correct copy to your agent. Your agent cannot bill the client (and you cannot be paid) until the voucher is turned in by you.

Most vouchers contain descriptions of the use that will be made of the pictures taken. Never permit a change to be made to that description. The use determines the rate and how much you are to be paid. Be certain that you know what the pictures will be used for. Never, never sign a blank model's or photo release under any circumstances. Use only the release given you by your agent. A signed blank release allows the holder to use your pictures for any purpose.

If you ever see your picture on a bus, a billboard, packaging or hangtags, or in a magazine anywhere in the world, including Europe or Asia, and feel that your voucher did not include such a use, contact your agency, no matter how much time has passed. You may be entitled to additional compensation, including damages for unauthorized use. Similarly, most vouchers limit the right to use your photo for a specific period of time, such as for one year. Use after that cut-off date entitles you to more money.

MODEL'S LIABILITY

When your agent accepts a booking for you, and you agree to do the shoot, a contract is created between you and the client. Models are independent contractors, not employees. If you are late or for some reason do not go to the booking without being excused by the client, the client will bill the agency for lost time on the set, which will include the time of the photographer, stylists, assistants, and the other models. You are legally obligated for those costs. Normally the agency will deduct all such charges from your compensation on other jobs, and such a provision is customarily found in the agency/model contract.

As an independent contractor, you are liable for your own federal and state income taxes, and normally the agency will not withhold them from your compensation. Once you finish a job, or leave an agency, you are not entitled to receive unemployment compensation. Agencies do not carry workmen's compensation insurance.

TWO

6

United States of America

I started interviewing people in New York for this book. Then I went around the world to interview agents in other fashion capitals. I returned to New York and talked to more agents, models, photographers, and hair and makeup artists. The pieces of the jigsaw finally came together here. Other American cities, however, merit attention because they offer excellent opportunities to models.

New York City

New York is the core of the modeling industry. Under the layers of glamour, expensive egos, and jet-set life-styles there is enormous organization, dedication, and incomparable *savoir-faire*.

There are about eighty agencies in the city for men, women, children, and parts models (models working specifically with eyes, lips, hands, legs, or other parts of the body). A top female model can make over $200,000 a year, and this does not include the superstars who make millions. A good male model can make $50,000 to $75,000 a year. Women are required to be 5'9" to 6'0" and over, with weight in proportion to height. The age range is sixteen to twenty-one, but there are exceptions at both ends of the scale. Several of today's superstars are over twenty-one.

Requirements for men are: height 6'0" to 6'2"; weight 165 to 170 pounds; measurements to fit a size 40 Regular or Long jacket, neck 15–15½, waist 30–32, shirt sleeve 33–35, and inseam 31"–34".

Agencies want experienced models with excellent portfolios, but they are always looking for new faces. Each agency has its own unique look. If you have it, they will take you on, test you, and do everything in their power to make you a success.

New York is a fast-paced city, but at least everyone speaks the same language, and there is an excellent inexpensive transportation system. This is a major plus for models who spend their days racing from one side of the city to the other.

Being on the cover of American *Vogue* is every model's dream, but the chances of achieving it are remote. Remuneration for doing this or any other cover assignment is very small, between $200 and $300. But once the word of a cover assignment reaches clients, photographers, and other agents, the model is an immediate success. Her agency's phones will ring constantly. The financial rewards can be astronomical.

Most New York agents send their models overseas, mainly to Paris and Milan. Foreign agents respect their New York colleagues and are eager to keep this international alliance profitable and happy. When agents send models to Europe they monitor their progress closely. The European agent strives for maximum exposure for the model, setting up appointments with photographers, editors, and clients. The end result is a portfolio of pictures and tear sheets that are fairly sure to guarantee work and financial success in New York. The bonus is the wealth of experience the model has acquired in Europe.

The agencies in New York are excellent. They are friendly, give outstanding service, and are looking for that new face that will be tomorrow's superstar. They all have testing boards and take 20 percent commission. The organization that sets the rules and guidelines is the International Model Managers Association (IMMA). To belong to IMMA one must be established as a model manager, have a voucher system and a head sheet, and have been in the business in New York for over a year.

Structured model agencies as we know them today began with John Robert Powers, a fascinating man who, after a brief spell as an actor and model, found himself spending more and more time acting as a liaison between photographers who needed models, and friends of his—aspiring actors and actresses—who were only too delighted to pose in front of a camera. As the demand for models grew, Powers realized that there was a genuine need for a structured agency that would represent the models fairly. He made history. In 1923, he started the world's first model agency in New York. Paulette Goddard, Barbara Stanwyck, Henry Fonda, Brian Donlevy, and Gene Tierney were among his first models. The John Robert Powers Agency was an enormous success and dominated the business for over a quarter of a century. By the late forties, Powers had turned his talents to writing, cosmetics, and a modeling school business. And another success story was beginning for a brilliant young woman whose name was to become world famous—Eileen Ford.

Ford Models

This agency is the most prestigious in the world. In my travels, I found that the name Eileen Ford is known by people not even remotely connected with the business. Eileen and her husband, Jerry, have carved out the top notch in the history of the profession. They started their agency in 1947 and made it the most successful on record. Eileen instinctively recognizes the potential for success. The girls she chooses are tall and sleek, with high cheekbones and a combination of beautiful features. If a girl has to rely on any one feature as a claim to fame she is not accepted. Jerry Ford handles the finances and public relations side of the business and is brilliant at both.

Eileen pulled no punches when I asked her for her advice to new models. She said: "Too many parents want to live vicariously through their children. They are all too eager to send them over to Europe like sugarplum fairies. Avarice will get these people nowhere but into trouble. A child is a precious thing—to treat it like a commodity is cruel."

She had this to say about young models going to Europe: "One fact you must face is that when a child is sent to Europe, she will receive no supervision. The super agents don't supervise—they don't have time. I am not talking about Switzerland or Germany. These countries are safe, and someone like Soni Ekvall at Model Team in Hamburg will take care of her models. To go to Europe a child must be very well adjusted. They are subject to temptations here, but these temptations are not handed out with a hand kiss and a gorgeous Italian accent."

Very young girls accepted by the Ford agency are invited to live with the Ford family while they are learning the business.

This agency is very diverse. In addition to the men's, women's, and children's divisions, there is: Ford/Classic Women (fashion and print for experienced models ages forty and over); Ford/Hands & Feet; Ford/Petite (height 5'3"–5'5", ages 18–21, size 6–8); Ford/Today's Women (fashion and print for experienced models ages 30–40); and Ford/12 Plus–Big Beauties (height 5'8" and over, ages 18–23, size 12–18).

In March 1991 the Ford agency opened Ford France in Paris (see chapter 12). Joe Hunter, executive vice president, told me: "American girls now feel that they have a safe haven in Paris."

Agency address: Ford Models Inc., 344 E. 59th Street, New York, NY 10022. Tel. (212) 753-6500.

Fran Rothchild and William (Bill) Weinberg are icons of the modeling industry. Fran co-founded the Wilhelmina Agency with the Dutch beauty Wilhelmina in 1967. When Wilhelmina died in 1980, Fran and Bill became joint owners. They are now retired from this agency.

Over the years Fran has seen thousands of models launch careers. Many have become superstars. We discussed the problems and misconceptions of new models. She said: "So many girls have no idea what is involved in establishing a career. They think that when they come to New York or go to Europe they will be on the cover of *Vogue* in a few weeks. If you stop to think about it, *Vogue* has twelve issues a year. Of these twelve covers three or four may be reserved for major actresses and stars like Liza Minnelli. This leaves seven or eight covers for all of the top models in the world. Kim Alexis had six or seven covers of *Vogue* in one year. Newcomers must know and accept these facts. They should also know that there are girls who make a lot of money but have never been seen on the cover of a magazine. These models are the bread and butter of the agencies. Above all it takes time to establish a career and make money."

Fran explained why it is necessary for new girls to go to Europe and why the European market is a significant factor in launching a career. "New models have to get tear sheets in order to put together a portfolio. The quickest way to do this is to go to Europe. There are many more opportunities there. Europe has more fashion magazines, and many of these are published with greater frequency. New York shoots today for a publication that will appear seven or eight months from now. Europe shoots today for a magazine that will come out in a month or so. I do not think, however, that models should go to Europe unless they are represented by a strong New York agent. There are matters they can't handle by themselves."

Bill Weinberg also has genuine concern for newcomers to the modeling profession both here and abroad. His answer to my question about advice for these young men and women was quick and serious: "Trust no one and be suspicious of everyone.'' He did not elaborate on this, but his words haunted me as I traveled around the world and met young people who had been betrayed by ''friends,'' or whose careers had floundered in the hands of unscrupulous agents.

Wilhelmina Model Agency

This is the third largest agency in the world. Its namesake, Wilhelmina, had an extraordinarily successful career as a model. Her equally successful career as an agent ended when she died at the age of forty, a victim of lung cancer.

It is now owned by Natasha Esch, an impressive young woman who took over from her father, Dieter Esch, in 1993. I met Natasha at her agency—an oasis of flowers and air-conditioning in sweltering mid-July New York! She told me: ''I had the advantage of having interned here at the agency during summer vacations from college, and basically knew everyone before I arrived. Models could relate to me because of my age. This was an advantage.'' Natasha advised: ''Parents must keep a level head. This business looks so glamorous. If your son or daughter wants to model, inquire about a good agency. Don't get involved with schemes that involve thousands of dollars for pictures or schools. It's not smart to waste money on a portfolio when you don't know what anyone is looking for. These scams take your money, stop the reputable agencies from finding the true talent we are looking for, and give our business a bad name. Send a couple of pictures—snapshots are fine—to the top New York agents, or a reputable agent in your home town. If they are interested, they will call you and take it from there. The industry is trying hard to make it very easy to inquire about this business in a legitimate way. The Ford, Elite, and Wilhelmina agencies hold nationwide contests. This is a very cheap way to find out if you are the face that is being sought after.''

The look for this agency is ''clean, healthy, young.'' The

age range is 14 to 50. Natasha said of the sophisticated division for older models: "This is a growing market. Baby boomers are getting older and there is a demand for that type of model." There are fashion, print, and runway divisions and also a very strong children's division.

Agency address: Wilhelmina Model Agency, 300 Park Avenue South, New York, NY 10010. Tel. (212) 473-0700. Fax (212) 473-3223.

Company

Company is a family-run, rapidly expanding business owned by Michael Flutie. The ratio of bookers to models is high, which means more attention can be given to individual careers. Michael said: "When a girl makes the decision to come to an agency like Company, it is like making the decision to go to a small private university that has a low student enrollment, an excellent staff, and excellent academic references versus a very large university with a huge staff and enrollment and an outstanding academic reputation. It is like choosing Vassar over Princeton or Yale. She won't get lost in the crowd, and there will be a lot of motivation and supervision."

There are several divisions at Company including film, television, and licensing divisions. The development division handles brand-new girls and models who have had up to two years of working experience. The management division is designed specifically to manage the careers of well-established models. "This is our superstar division. We have eight girls who work internationally and make a great deal of money. Our goal is to lay the foundation for a long, successful career in the development stage and then motivate and enable girls to move up into the management division."

We discussed age requirements. Michael said: "We don't encourage anyone to move to New York full-time until they have finished high school. Education is a very important criteria with us. I don't think clients focus on how old a girl is as long as she is fresh-looking, has good skin, is well-established, and has a strong editorial book. I think a girl can work until she is thirty-five. However, it is too late to start a career at twenty-two."

Company now has an agency in Paris.

Michael reiterated the constantly recurring theme that a model should have a New York agent prior to going to Europe or any foreign country.

"I care very much about what happens to our youth, especially the people who enter this business. It is unfortunate that some of our young athletes and models fall into the hands of people pretending to be experts. Some fail not because of their lack of ability but because of these people. A model should seek out the people in the business who have put strong emphasis on being honest and legitimate."

Agency address: Company, 270 Lafayette St., Suite 1400, New York, NY 10012. Tel. (212) 226-7000. Fax (212) 226-9791.

Foster-Fell

Englishman Jeremy Foster-Fell, the owner, discussed his agency and changes in the industry in the last few years. "My emphasis is still fashion, but it is also commercial. These days the two overlap. We are also seeing older women in the business. The other day we booked a seventy-year-old for a cosmetic commercial. We had sent a fifty-year-old and were told she wasn't old enough! This would never have happened ten or fifteen years ago. The marketing people are beginning to realize that they have to make specific products for specific age groups and that teenagers are not the major money spenders in America." I asked Jeremy for his views on the multimillion-dollar contracts signed by top models. He said: "In twenty-five years we have come from a relatively small business to a multimillion-dollar industry. When someone is responsible for over three hundred million dollars worth of sales of a product, this is a very important spokesperson. You are looking at enormous amounts of sales tied to somebody's face, and I think they are underpaid—which is a highly controversial position.''

Agency address: Foster-Fell, 36 East 23rd Street, New York, NY 10010. Tel. (212) 353-0300. Fax (212) 353-0160.

Zoli

Rosmarie Chalem, who is Swiss, came to Zoli in 1982. She is the director of the women's division. Rosmarie is interested in girls who are at least 5′9″ tall and who are between the ages of fifteen and twenty. She has this advice for newcomers to the business: ''If a young girl has the potential, and a good head on her shoulders, this can be a very nice profession for her. From the very beginning she has to realize that it takes a long time to become a good model. It rarely happens overnight. When success does come she must not let it change her. We do send girls to Europe, but I warn them to be careful—especially in Milan. I only work with agents I can trust.''

Zoli has been in existence for over twenty-two years. It has fashion, editorial, advertising, and television divisions. Open calls are held for women on Tuesdays and Thursdays between 11 A.M. and 12 noon.

The men's division has fifty models and has a strong worldwide reputation. Minimum height requirement is 6′0″ and the age range is seventeen to fifty-five. Roseanne Vecchione, who heads this division, came to Zoli four years ago, having spent fifteen years in the same division at Wilhelmina Models. We discussed the long career span enjoyed by male models. Roseanne explained: ''There is much more leeway with men. They don't have to be concerned with face wrinkles. In fact, we find that wrinkles give them more appeal. When they are being photographed the lighting doesn't have to be perfect. If it is a bit shadowy or dark, it lends toward masculinity. Women have to have everything perfect. Men are lucky; they have very long careers. Our most prestigious models don't base themselves in one market, they make the circuit—Milan, Paris, London. However, this is an industry where women make much more money than men. There are more fashion magazines and more products for women and women spend more money on all of these."

We discussed other aspects of modeling careers for men and the changes that have taken place in the last few years. Roseanne said: "It has become much more acceptable for a man to become a model. In Italy there are a lot of fashion magazines for men who study them and gear their style to that trend. Here, there are fewer magazines, but men are starting to read about fashion and to take a greater interest in what they wear. It is becoming acceptable for men to be interested in fashion.

"The biggest change I have seen in the last few years is the look for male models. It used to be a street-type look: plain, unusual, sultry. Now the style is more upscale. A rich look. A Cary Grant style. I like this."

Open calls for the men's division are held Monday through Friday from 10:30 to 11 A.M.

Agency address: Zoli, 3 W. 18th Street, New York, NY 10011. Tel. (212) 242-1500. Fax (212) 242-7505.

Elite Model Management

John Casablancas, the dynamic force behind the Elite agency, was born in New York of wealthy Spanish parents. He was educated in Switzerland and traveled extensively in Europe and South America. In 1971, after a trial-and-error period, he started his modeling empire in Paris with the opening of Elite—an agency for the crème de la crème, the model superstars. L'Agence, an agency for grooming new talent, followed. In 1977 he fused his European *savoir-vivre* with his acquired American *savoir-faire* and exploded onto the American scene. He opened an Elite agency in New York to the chagrin of his competitors. John Casablancas's rise to fame was rapid and his success phenomenal. Today he has the largest modeling network in the world. His "Look of the Year" model contest is the largest international model search.

Elite is always looking for new models. Height requirement is 5′9″ (min.) and the age range is sixteen to twenty years. If you have a well-proportioned body, a classic face, a sparkling personality, and an elegant but not too sophisticated style you could be right for this agency.

Agency address: 111 E. 22nd Street, New York, NY 10010. Tel. (212) 529-9700. Fax (212) 475-1332.

IMG Models

Started in February 1987, IMG Models has become one of New York's leading agencies. It is a division of International Management Group, the sports management corporation that handles the commercial careers of Bjorn Borg, Martina Navratilova, and other superstars of the sports world. Owned by Mark Mc-Cormack, IMG has produced a crop of models that includes Julie Anderson, Carrie Johnson, Niki Taylor, and Lauren Hutton.

I asked Leah McCloskey, director of scouting and talent development, what she looks for in a model. She said: "I look for an individual who has the qualifications and ability to work in a high-fashion market and who can be developed on a completely different level. The trend is getting much more toward larger than life personalities. The days of a girl being only meek and quiet but beautiful and great in front of a camera are close to the end. Though the still photography aspect will remain important, models will have to be able to make the transition to talking on camera and being a personality as well. Models have become of enormous interest to the public. They are better known than some actors and actresses. They are the key interest in the public eye."

Agency address: IMG Models, 170 Fifth Avenue, 10th Floor, New York, NY 10010. Tel. (212) 627-0400. Fax (212) 627-4992.

Margaret Models Inc.

This is a family-run agency that opened in 1988. Margaret Matuka, for whom the agency is named, is the mother of two immensely successful models: Maggie Woods, who is the director of scouting and head of the women's division, and Kim Matuka, who runs the children's division. During an interview Kim explained: "We have been on both sides of this business and know what it is like to go on castings. We can relate to models. We don't accept a lot of girls [the agency has about thirty] but those we do accept, we push beyond belief. The family believes that careers can be started in New York, that a girl can become a super model here without going to Europe."

Age range for the women's division is twelve—the agency has 5'9" Liza, a gorgeous Russian super model—to twenty-four. There is a men's division for commercials and print. The petite division formed in 1994 in partnership with Fernando Casablancas is called Get Real. Here the requirements are: girls aged fourteen to twenty-two; height 5'4" to 5'9"; fresh classic beauty; thin (hips maximum 34"); beautiful skin and a great smile.

Agency address: Margaret Models Inc., 276 Fifth Avenue, Suite 1001, New York, NY 10001. Tel. (212) 532-6005. Fax (212) 643-1794.

BOSS

BOSS opened its doors in New York in 1988 (and in London in 1992). Among its twenty women is superstar Amber Valletta. The seventy-five-strong men's division includes top male model Marcus Schenkenberg. David Bosman, the president, is English and a former fashion photographer and model. He told me: "Five of our girls represent new talent, the remaining fifteen are established superstars. We are looking for girls with personality as well as looks. Having just a pretty face doesn't quite cut it anymore." He added: "We are a management agency, but a management agency that understands fashion as opposed to just being in the fashion business."

Agency address: BOSS, 317 W. 13th Street, New York, NY 10014. Tel. (212) 242-2444.

Click Models

Owned by Frances Grill, this agency has been going strong since 1979. It has a men's division, as well as fashion, print, and television departments. Minimum height requirement for women is 5'8"; age: fourteen to twenty-two.

Agency address: Click Models, 881 Seventh Avenue, New York, NY 10019. Tel. (212) 315-2200.

Partners

Partners arrived in New York and Paris on September 1, 1993. David Bonnouvrier is the president and director of the women's division; Camilla Cassels-Smith directs the men's division. Discussing the male model market, Camilla said: "There is no comparison to the women's market. There is less work and less money. However, there are some male models who make $500,000 annually." Describing the look for women, she continues: "Our true search is for the girl who will be high editorial, someone a particular photographer is going to be very interested in. A girl may walk in, and we'll say to ourselves, Steven Meisel or Bruce Weber would really like her. We then try to cultivate an image we can promote for her. Partners is well connected internationally, and the owners and staff are gracious.

Agency address: Partners, 415 W. Broadway, New York, NY (212) 966-0090. Fax (212) 966-4567.

Paris/USA Models

Opened in 1987, Paris/USA is owned by Louise Roberts, a model agent for over thirty years, and Douglas Asch, who has been an agent for eleven years. They represent between forty and fifty models. Minimum height requirement for women is 5'9" and for men 6'0".

I asked Douglas for his views on the modeling profession today. He said: "It is not enough for a girl to be pretty. She must be more disciplined, more professional, and have greater personality and style than ever before. The shrinking world economy and the ever-increasing influx of new models has made it much more difficult for a model's career to get started. The business has polarized in the last few years. More young girls are struggling to get established and on the other end of the spectrum there are the superstars who are used over and over again by the top people all over the world. I think that the middle ground has gone."

I asked Douglas if a new model could start her career in New York without first going to Europe. He replied: "At this agency we believe that a girl with top potential can get started in New York. We feel that having had experience here she will be more professional, have a better knowledge of the business, and therefore get more out of the opportunities in Europe. This is our personal belief; it is certainly not the way other agents feel."

The agency holds open interviews Thursdays from 5 to 6 P.M.

Agency address: 470 Park Avenue South, Room 1704, New York, NY 10016. Tel. (212) 683-9040. Fax (212) 683-0946.

Nytro

This agency (formerly Manner) is exclusively for men. President Jan Gonet draws on eighteen years' experience with the world's top agencies to discuss the male modeling business.

"It's in a state of flux. There are too many models and not enough jobs. Only the best are working. There is confusion as to what is popular and what is not. This is a very serious business. Men must be dedicated and behave in a professional manner. Looks, height, and personality are important. For Nytro, I look for someone who is strong and masculine; someone who can create an image and go beyond the obvious when they are in front of a camera.

Agency address: Nytro, 134 Spring Street, New York, NY 10012. Tel. (212) 219-2300. Fax (212) 219-3714.

Formation and FM²

Founder of and mastermind behind these agencies is Karol Hodges, ably assisted by head booker Tony Iuffredo. Karol is one of the most sought-after fit models (a fit model is one who has clothing designed and fitted to her measurements) on Seventh Avenue. Realizing the need for this type of model, she started FM², which represents men and women as well as photographers, makeup artists, and stylists. Formation is her very successful talent agency.

Agency address: 156 Fifth Avenue, Suite 515, New York, NY 10010. Tel. (212) 675-7037. Fax (212) 675-7642.

HV Models/Maxx Men

Heinz Vollenweider, a Swiss, owns both agencies, which were opened in 1983 and 1990 respectively. HV Models is the women's division. Models must be at least 5'8" tall and have a young, beautiful, fresh look. Age range is sixteen to twenty-three. Maxx Men concentrates on men who can bridge the gap from editorial to advertising. Minimum height requirement is 6'0". Suit size is 40 Regular. Age range is eighteen to thirty-five.

Address for both agencies: 30 East 20th Street, New York, NY 10003. Tel. (212) 228-0300 (HV Models); (212) 228-0278 (Maxx Men). Fax (212) 228-0438.

Pauline's Model Management

This delightful agency was opened in August 1984 by Canadian-born Pauline Bernatchez. Pauline, who originally modeled in Paris, has an agency there also. There are fifty girls at the New York connection. Height requirements are 5'9" to 6'1" and the age range is fifteen to twenty-three. Pauline's has fashion, print, and television divisions.

Agency address: Pauline's Model Management, 379 W. Broadway, New York, NY 10012. Tel. (212) 941-6000.

Plus Models/Swift Kids

Owned by Pat Swift, this agency is dedicated to large-size and petite women and children. It handles fashion, print, and runway work.

Agency address: 49 W. 37th Street, New York, NY 10018. Tel. (212) 997-1785. Fax (212) 302-4375.

Gilla Roos

This agency handles commercial and print work. There is no fashion division. All types of models are listed as there is no height, age, weight, or size requirement.

Agency address: Gilla Roos, 16 W. 22nd Street, New York, NY 10010. Tel. (212) 727-7820.

Chicago

Chicago was not what I had expected. Hollywood had distorted my vision! I thought machine-gun-toting gangsters would lurk on every corner. (Well, I did see a gangster tour advertised!) As in every big city there is a crime problem and wandering the streets at night is not advisable. But Chicago is basically a happy, friendly city with beautiful Lake Michigan shimmering in the center.

For models, Chicago is a good balance—a big city with big-city opportunities and a small town with small-town friendliness. It is the second largest market in the country and offers a wide range of modeling. Here you will find print, high fashion, run-way, showroom, television, catalog, and fitting work. There is work for the perfect size model, as well as large sizes, petites, juniors, and children, plus hand and foot models. There is also a strong male market. And there is a constant flow of models to and from Europe and Japan.

The fashion industry in Chicago has seen many changes in recent years as a result of the Sears pull-out and the financial failure of many catalog houses. Catalogs formerly provided most of the work in Chicago, but now the emphasis has shifted to other areas. However, Chicago is still a good city in which to begin a modeling career. Agents are willing to work with new faces to develop them for their own agencies as well as other markets. Yet, as in every other big market, the competition is strong and professionalism and patience are essential.

Elite Chicago Model Management

Elite Chicago is a high-fashion agency representing men and women. Height for women is 5'9", with some exceptions; for men, 6'0".

Agency address: 212 W. Superior #406, Chicago, IL 60610. Tel. (312) 943-3226. Fax (312) 943-2590.

Arlene Wilson Management

Energetic, with an excellent staff, Arlene Wilson is a full-service agency for men, women, children, plus-sizes, and petites. Height requirement is 5′9″ to 5′10″ (5′8″ occasionally) for women; 5′11″ to 6′0″ for men. Discussing the Chicago market, director Kevin Menard explained: "Everything in the Midwest is upscale. Clients are still paying $1500-a-day rates but they want high-caliber models. When models come through town with strong books, they get the lion's share of the work. The Asian and Hispanic markets are expanding rapidly. Chicago is a very diverse town."

Agency address: Arlene Wilson Management, 430 West Erie, Suite 210, Chicago, IL 60610. Tel. (312) 573-0200. Fax (312) 573-0046.

David and Lee Models

Lee Whitfield and her daughters Robin and Noelle (both graphic designers) and a wonderful staff run this agency. Lee told me: "We look for young models in their teens to twenty-two. Girls must be 5′9″ to 5′10″ and guys 6′0″ to 6′1″. We take new people as well as established models. I love to get careers started. If we are to have a future, we must always be looking for that new face.

Agency address: David and Lee Models, 70 W. Hubbard, Chicago, IL 60610. Tel. (312) 661-0500. Fax (312) 661-0760.

Susanne's A-Plus Talent Agency

After ten successful years with her own agency, Susanne Johnson merged Susanne Johnson Talent with A-Plus Talent (Sharon Wottrich, president) to meet the needs of a diversifying industry. The combined reputations and experience of these two businesses have made the agency a major force in the city. Discussing the merger, Susanne told me: "In 1985 you could run an agency just on fashion, but today in Chicago you can't do that. By joining our two agencies we have been able to broaden our range tremendously. We have print, commercial, television, film, and convention divisions, and very strong children's and large size divisions."

Agency address: 108 W. Oak, Chicago, IL 60610. Tel. (312) 943-8315. Fax (312) 943-9751.

Aria Models

Long-time agent and scout Marie Anderson, who discovered Cindy Crawford, is part owner of Aria Models, one of the newer agencies. Marie said: "It's for men and women and has every division but runway and animals!"

Agency address: Aria Models, 1017 W. Washington, Suite 2A, Chicago, IL 60607. Tel. (312) 243-9400. Fax (312) 243-9020.

Dallas

Dallas is a refined city renowned for its beautiful women. The modeling industry here has grown rapidly in the last five years, and there are over thirty model agencies in the city. All categories of modeling are represented and it is a good market for male models.

Kim Dawson Agency

The first model agency in Dallas was opened in 1961 by Kim Dawson. One of the first international models, Kim started her career with the John Robert Powers agency in New York. She was one of the first American girls to model the Collections for the famous couture houses in Paris. Kim told me: "There were no agencies in Paris at that time. We just made calls on the couture houses. They considered it a great status symbol to have an American model wear their clothes." When she returned to the United States and Dallas, she opened her own agency, the Kim Dawson Agency. The business is a family affair—Kim's husband, George, a photographer, and daughter Lisa, who has also modeled in Paris, are actively involved.

Kim pays great attention to her models' welfare and progress. She is very concerned about the large number of girls who go into the modeling profession and she is particularly concerned about the models who go to Europe. "The modeling profession has had so much publicity in recent years that we have an overwhelming load of models in every market in the world—and there are not that many markets. The media hype has resulted in mothers who feel that their daughters just have to be part of this business. So often when a girl goes to Europe, it is the mother's dream that has come true and not necessarily the child's."

Kim is very direct when talking to models and their mothers about the business in Europe. She told me: "I stress that Europe is the beginning of a nightmare for many children—a lot of these young women are more child than adult. I tell them they are going to a culture that has a lot to do with drugs and sex. I am very honest with them because I have had too many girls come back to tell me horror stories of their experiences. If young people are well informed and well prepared and if they realize that their whole life is more important than the next five years, they will approach the business with a totally different attitude." On her life in the industry, Kim says: "It is a business to which I am enormously grateful. I have made a career in Dallas and my agency has made a difference in Dallas."

Kim's daughter and agency director, Lisa Dawson, draws on her experience as an international model to pass on this advice to newcomers: "New girls have to be adaptable. When they go to Europe if they are told to cut their hair, or to use less makeup, they must follow instructions. Many girls from provincial markets will cry and get upset when they are asked to change their look. We can test them here and put together a portfolio. But if they can work and get tear sheets in Europe, they will do so much better when they come back."

The Kim Dawson Agency also has divisions for men and children. All categories of modeling are represented.

Agency address: 2300 Stemmons Freeway, Dallas, TX 75258. Tel. (214) 638-2414. Fax (214) 638-7567.

Page Parkes Model's Rep

Page Parkes brought an international flair to the modeling industry in Dallas and Houston. She went to school in London and attended the American School of Fine Arts in Paris. In Europe she scouted for models for the Dallas market.

In 1979 Page and her business partner, Rachel Duran, opened the Page Parkes Center of Modeling in Houston, a testing and training facility for new models. This was followed by the InterMedia Model and Talent Agency, which established models in the local Houston market. The two women then took their expertise to Dallas, where they started the Page Parkes Model's Rep, an agency designed exclusively for models with international experience. Page told me: "In Dallas we look for girls with special features. They must be at least 5'9", have beauty, and have had editorial experience on an international level. Our goal is to make them stars." Model's Rep, which now has a sister agency in Miami, provides personal service and representation for a select group of high-income models. It also ensures a high standard of professionalism for clients.

Agency address: 3131 McKinney, Suite 430, Dallas, TX 75204. Tel. (214) 871-9003. Fax (214) 871-0044.

Houston

This is a growing market and an ideal place for male and female models to launch their careers. All aspects of modeling are covered by twenty-five agencies.

Page Parkes Center of Modeling is located at 5353 W. Alabama—#220, Houston, TX 77056. Tel. (713) 622-7171. Fax (713) 622-4918.

The InterMedia Models and Talent Agency is at 5353 W. Alabama—#222, Houston, TX 77056. Tel. (713) 622-8282. Fax (713) 622-4918.

Los Angeles

Los Angeles is one of the world's most competitive markets for agents and models. Many new agencies have failed recently as a result of major financial problems in the fashion industry. There is a superabundance of models, and the majority have all the necessary qualifications. The big allure is the movie industry and the opportunities for television. Top models who can demand and receive big booking fees in New York often prefer to make Los Angeles their base in the hope that they will make the overnight, lucrative leap from model to movie star or celebrity. In the meantime an established model can get direct bookings for assignments in Milan, Paris, Germany, London, Japan, and Australia. An average working model can earn between $30,000 and $60,000 a year.

There is strong competition for male models. Los Angeles abounds with male actors who have had successful modeling careers in New York, Paris, and Milan.

Los Angeles is a good place for a model to begin but on a

small scale. Clients are conservative and won't take the chance of using a new model for a big campaign. Gerard Bisignano has experience as an international model and agent. He told me: "In Europe or New York people will take the gamble with a new face because they want to be able to say 'I discovered this person.' Here it is very rare that a model will take off and make money quickly. Clients want models with good portfolios. A model can start in L.A. but then he or she has to go to Europe or New York for experience. When they are more competitive they can come back here to work."

Gerard is concerned about the moral welfare of young people who choose modeling as a career. "In any industry where there is youth, beauty, and a lot of money to be made there is certainly great room for abuse. It is important that parents give their children a long-term spiritual foundation, with strong moral principles and a good sense of self-worth. With this type of background young people will realize that compromising their values is not the way to achieve success. If an agent suggests a moral compromise, a model will know that he or she is at the wrong agency."

Wilhelmina Models

Wilhelmina Models is owned by the parent company, Wilhelmina Model Agency of New York, and has been in Los Angeles for fifteen years. Co-directors are Terry Hinckley and Margot Law. The agency will take existing models with working experience at many different ages. A brand-new girl cannot be older than twenty, and a new male model must be under twenty-five. This is a high-fashion agency and while the minimum height for high-fashion models is normally 5'9", this agency will make an exception and take a girl who is 5'8" if she is special. Male models are 6'0" to 6'3".

Agency address: Wilhelmina Models, 8383 Wilshire Blvd., Beverly Hills, CA 90211. Tel. (213) 655-0909.

Hero Model Management

An exclusively men's agency, the required height is 6'0" and the age, seventeen and over. Model agent Ken Steckla told me: "Male models have to be prepared to travel a lot, in this country and overseas. We have many foreign clients—at least those not scared away by fire, riots, earthquakes, and mudslides!" Hero looks for men who can do newspaper, catalog, and television work as well as advertise a wide range of products, with emphasis on swimwear and athletics. The agency has fashion, print, music, and television divisions. It is always interested in new faces.

Agency address: Hero Model Management, 9255 Sunset Blvd., Suite 727, Los Angeles, CA 90069. Tel. (310) 285-0508. Fax (310) 285-0965.

Fontaine Model Agency

This is one of five agencies owned by Judy Fontaine. "We represent models ranging from new faces to superstars. The look in California is very healthy, fresh, and body-conscious. Los Angeles is a fashion city. We couldn't be in business without fashion. We consider swimwear fashion. All of the major swimsuit companies are here. They supply 250 million people in this country," she said.

The Fontaine Agency represents two hundred models ages sixteen and over. Minimum height is 5'7".

(See also Fontaine Kids, chapter 20.)

Agency address: 9255 Sunset Blvd., Los Angeles, CA 90069. Tel. (310) 285-0545. Fax (310) 285-9053.

LA Models (Also LA Talent and LA Kids)

Owned by Heinz Holba, LA Models was opened in 1984 and has divisions for men, women, and children. Vice President

Patsy Beattie has had twenty years of experience in the business, and had these comments on the modeling and fashion industries: "I have seen major changes in the entire business, especially through corporate mergers and department store bankruptcies. There will have to be some kind of evolution in retailing that will affect the modeling industry in the future." Ages range from five to sixty.

Agency address: LA Models, 8335 Sunset Boulevard, 2nd Floor, Los Angeles, CA 90069. Tel. (213) 656-9572. Fax (213) 656-0489.

Nina Blanchard Agency

Nina Blanchard is the First Lady of the industry on the West Coast. Nina's original ambition was to be an actress and she went to New York to achieve this goal. "When I knew I could not be a Joanne Woodward, I gave up the idea. I'm glad I realized this when I did, otherwise I would still be a waitress in New York hoping to become an actress." Nina has this advice for young models and actors: "For the last thirty-eight years I have heard people say they are insecure. *Everyone* is insecure—if you are not insecure, you are dead! Don't drain your emotional energy on negative thinking or anger. Spend it on things that matter. Use your emotional energy to do something with yourself." This agency has open calls every day from 2:30 P.M. to 3:30 P.M.

Agency address: Nina Blanchard Agency, 957 Cole Avenue, Los Angeles, CA 90038. Tel. (213) 462-7274.

BAMM

This stands for Bill Arndt Model Management. Bill, who has been in the business for many years, started BAMM in 1992. He has been a strong advocate of men in the modeling world and has always believed that a male model's career has the same respectability as that of a female model's. He has been responsible for boosting this part of the industry. Ages range from eighteen to forty.

Agency address: BAMM, 8609 Sherwood Drive, West Hollywood, CA 90069. Tel. (310) 652-6252.

C' La Vie Model and Talent Agency

C' La Vie is an abbreviation of the French expression *c'est la vie*. The agency, whose president is Jean-Marc Carré, has strong international connections. There are television, editorial, catalog, and commercial print divisions. Director Steve Landry adds: "We also have 'kids,' starting at kindergarten, and grandparents."

Agency address: C' La Vie, 7507 Sunset Blvd., Suite 201, Los Angeles, CA 90046. Tel. (213) 969-0541. Fax (213) 969-0401.

Elite/L.A.

Elite/L.A. opened in 1979 as the West Coast headquarters for the giant Elite Model Management Corporation in New York. With a worldwide network of model agencies at its disposal this agency can find the appropriate markets for all of its models. It has a small, selective men's division and represents models for film, print, catalog, and television work.

Agency address: Elite/L.A., 9255 Sunset Boulevard, Los Angeles, CA 90069. Tel. (213) 274-9395.

There are other good agencies in Los Angeles. Check the city telephone directory for listings.

San Francisco

When the weather is cold in Europe and New York, clients find San Francisco a perfect location because of its climate and beautiful scenery.

Stars

Lynn Claxon, owner of the very successful Stars agency, had this to say about the market: "San Francisco is an ideal place for a model to get her feet wet and to get used to living away from home for the first time. It is smaller and more personal than New York and we have excellent photographers here. Although this is mainly an advertising town, there is a broad spectrum of work that includes fashion, theater, and television."

Lynn's husband Colin, who co-owns the agency, is an entertainment attorney whose expertise is invaluable when dealing with the legal rights of models here and overseas (see chapter 5).

As parents, the Claxons relate to the concern of other parents whose daughters are starting careers away from home. Lynn says, "We make every effort to brief them on what they must expect in this business. We are particularly concerned about girls who have never been to Europe before. We tell them what they should and shouldn't do and what to beware of. As their mother agent we make sure that we deal with only the most reputable agents and we keep abreast of what is happening within the business around the world. Stars is based on hard work and a very high standard of integrity." Very young girls stay with the Claxons at their home.

Stars is very much a family business. The Claxon's daughter Kristin is director of fashion and son Scott is in charge of new faces and scouting, here and abroad.

Stars has recently added Jimmy Grimmé (formerly the Grimmé Agency) and his Grimmé men to its fashion division.

Height requirement for girls is 5'8" minimum and the age requirement is twelve to twenty-one. Men must be 6'0" or over. Stars provides accommodations for new models and advances rent.

Agency address: Stars, 777 Davis Street, San Francisco, CA 94111. Tel. (415) 421-6272. Fax (415) 421-7620.

City Model Management and Mitchell Model Management are agencies with excellent reputations. For other listings check the telephone directory.

Seattle

Seattle is a significant scouting ground for agents from all over the world. I asked many of them why the Pacific Northwest attracted such attention. The consensus of opinion was that the beautiful climate and Scandinavian influence produced tall, healthy, strikingly beautiful girls who have "the clearest skin in the world."

This is a very friendly community and there is great rapport between clients and models. There is a lot of fashion show work here as well as catalog, advertising, and television. Models can also work in Los Angeles and San Francisco, which means they can work three markets at one time.

Seattle Models Guild

Owned by Joanne Meyers, a former international model, the agency has about fifty models whose ages range from nineteen to fifty. There is a large men's division here, and a couple of petite models are also represented. A model's career span is longer in Seattle. When models have worked internationally they can return and work for a considerably longer period than in other cities.

Agency address: Seattle Models Guild, 1809 Seventh Avenue, Seattle, WA 98101. Tel. (206) 622-1406.

There are several reputable agencies and modeling schools in the area. This city is an ideal place to learn about the modeling profession and launch a career. It has excellent liaisons with other American agencies and with top foreign agents.

Atlanta

L'Agence

Atlanta is a young, aggressive, steadily growing market with many good agencies. One of them is L'Agence, whose president is tall, good-looking Mark Cook. Mark and his mother, Gretta Cook, who is also his partner, run a highly organized international business. His sister, Senia, owns L'Agence in Miami. More recently the family opened the agency Class in Rio de Janeiro, Brazil, and Mark is considering Istanbul as a future market. I asked him about these exciting ventures. He told me: "Brazil is not established with its own models. Clients fly in models from abroad. Brazil has beautiful scenery, excellent photographers, and its own issues of *Harper's Bazaar, Vogue, Elle,* and Chinese *Elle.* A model can have tear sheets within a month and a complete portfolio suitable for the New York market within two months. This is not a money market, however, because of the soaring inflation rate. I am considering opening an agency in Istanbul because clients are always looking for new locations. They get a bit tired of Paris and Milan."

Of his home base, Mark said: "Atlanta is an easy transition for girls from the southeastern United States who plan eventually to work in New York or Europe."

L'Agence is a high-fashion agency that also does catalog and television work. Mark deals with agents in New York,

California, Chicago, and Europe. Describing the type of model represented by his agency, he told me: "The look for women is fresh, tall, and beautiful. Height requirement is 5'8" to 5'11". New models must be under twenty-one years of age unless they have been well established in another market. The look for men is clean-cut, athletic, and they must have very good bodies. They should be aged eighteen and over. Height requirement is 6'0" to 6'2" and the size for men is 40 Regular to 40 Long."

L'Agence also represents large-size models (size 14 and over) and petites. Mark said: "We have noticed a definite growth in the petite market in the last six months. In order to do well in the business, a petite model must be excellent. She must have good hands and feet, a good lingerie body, and an incredible face. A girl can be 5'9" and a fairly good model, and still make money. But a model who is 5'6" or less has to have a lot going for her."

Agency address: L'Agence, 12 Perimeter Center E.—Suite 2624, Atlanta, GA 30346. Tel. (404) 396-9015.

The Chez Group

This thriving business is the result of the experience and effort of owner Shay Griffin. Shay is a former model and has a good perspective of the industry. Her agency has print, commercial, casting, and trade show divisions and an active film division. Speaking about Atlanta, Shay explained: "Atlanta is an international city and consequently our business is becoming more and more international. There is also quite a good male model market here."

Agency address: The Chez Group, 1776 Peachtree Road, N.W. Suite 434, South Tower, Atlanta, GA 30309. Tel. (404) 873-1215. Fax (404) 874-7532.

Serendipity Models International, Inc.

This full-service agency is located in the heart of Atlanta's trendy Buckhead at 550 Pharr Road, Suite 220, Atlanta, GA 30305. Tel. (404) 237-4040. Fax (404) 231-4335.

Take time to check out other reputable agencies in Atlanta. A full range of modeling is available through them.

Miami

A sunny coastline, superb models, agencies that provide a full range of facilities, and worldwide publicity from television and film have contributed to Miami's rise from regional to international status. Clients from France, Italy, and Germany shoot catalog and print work in the area for six to nine months a year, making this region the largest market for fashion photography in the country.

Michele Pommier Models

Husband-and-wife team Michele Pommier and Peter Diel, who own Michele Pommier Models Inc., have played a significant part in Miami's success story. Michele has had over twenty years in the business as an international model (she was with the Ford agency) and agent. Peter is a computer whiz who has computerized the business to the extent that they know what is happening in the modeling industry ''all day, every day, all over the world.'' Together they have wooed and won impressive European accounts by anticipating the immediate needs of foreign directors, photographers, and film crews.

Models at this agency are over 5′8″ tall and have a young,

classic look. Male models must be 6′0″ tall. The agency has the largest children's division in the southeast.

I asked Michele what advice she would give aspiring models. She told me: "Modeling is a serious business. It is not a world playground. You can make good money if you are a true professional. Keep good hours. Leave partying for the weekends. Listen to someone you trust in the business—preferably your agent. Remember what your mom and dad taught you. If someone approaches you with drugs or improper suggestions—*just say no!*"

Agency address: Michele Pommier Models Inc., 1126 Ocean Drive, Miami Beach, FL 33139. Tel. (305) 667-8710.

Agencies in the Miami and Fort Lauderdale areas are competitive and offer excellent representation. Among these are:

L'Agence, 1220 Collins Avenue, Miami Beach, FL 33139. Tel. (305) 672-0804. Fax (305) 672-4250.
Page Parkes Model's Rep, 660 Ocean Drive, Miami Beach, FL 33139. Tel. (305) 672-4869. Fax (305) 672-1137. The rapidly growing Miami connection of the Dallas agency.
Irene Marie Inc., 728 Ocean Drive, Miami Beach, FL 33139. Tel. (305) 672-2929. Fax (305) 674-1342. A strong international agency.

The Ford, Elite, and Next agencies in New York are represented in Miami.

Tampa, Orlando, and Brevard County

These are local markets, and they illustrate how young boys or girls who dream of becoming models can achieve this goal provided they have potential and a good local agent. In winter clients from Canada and Europe come for the warm climate and beautiful settings this area offers. Universal Studios opened in Orlando in 1988 and began shooting as soon as sets were ready. Other film companies produce films here. The Disney Corporation provides a constant source of print and television commercial work for local talent.

Dott Burns Model and Talent Agency

One of the prime figures behind the international spotlight in Florida is Dott Burns, who opened her agency in Tampa in 1970. Dott is a remarkable woman who has a great sense of humor and an indomitable spirit. She has helped put Florida on the map as the third state in the nation for film work. She was the mainspring behind legislation that requires all agents in Florida to be licensed by the state. Explaining why she spent four years trying to get this bill passed, she said: "There were one hundred unqualified people acting as agents in Florida. There were no rules and there was no discipline. Bona fide agents and talent suffered as a result. This bill got rid of the scams and rip-offs."

Dott was a successful model and fashion illustrator in New York before coming to Tampa to be married. She had a daughter, Kim (now a wife, mother, and actress), and later began a career in television. This ended abruptly when a serious illness brought her close to death and confined her to a wheelchair. "One never knows what is going to happen in life. For this reason a model should always be prepared to do something else—to have an alternative means of making a living."

Her agency has been extremely successful. She discovered superstar model Jaci Adams. Dott said: "I saw Jaci in a shopping mall and gave her my card. I asked her to send me some photographs and she told me she didn't have any. I arranged for a couple of photographic sessions. I sent her to Eileen Ford in New York. She did some testing, came back to Tampa, and then went to Europe. She was on the cover of every magazine there. She came back to the U.S. and landed a very lucrative contract. She was a superstar. Jaci is exceptional. She is very beautiful, very stable, and really knows what she is doing. Not many girls have this combination. I am really careful that the girls I send to Europe are well balanced emotionally, as well as having all of the other qualifications.'' Dott says she probably would not be in the business today if it were not for the friendship and support of top agent Eileen Ford. ''About eight years ago, I was feeling discouraged and didn't think I could continue in the business. Eileen wrote me a scorching letter telling me to get my act together, that she expected more from me than to think of quitting. I felt that if a woman of her standing thought I could make it, then I would. And I did. Eileen is a great lady.''

Agency address: Dott Burns Talent Agency, 478 Severn Avenue, Tampa, FL 33606. Tel. (813) 251-5882. Fax (813) 253-2363.

Other Tampa agencies include:

Berg Talent Agency, 1115 Himes Avenue N., Tampa 33614. Tel. (813) 877-5533. Fax (813) 877-6012.
Trends Model Talent Inc., 2900 E. 7th Avenue, Tampa, FL 33605. Tel. (813) 248-4008.
John Casablancas Center, 5215 W. Laurel Street, Suite 203, Tampa, FL 33607. Tel. (813) 289-8564.
Avance Model/Talent Agency, 406 N. Reo Street, Tampa, FL 33609. Tel. (813) 289-9816.

Agencies in Orlando include:

The Cassandra Bailey Talent Agency, 513 W. Colonial Drive, Suite 6, Orlando, FL 32804. Tel. (407) 423-7872. Fax (407) 872-0559.
The Christensen Group, 114D Park Avenue S., Winter Park, FL 32789. Tel. (407) 628-8803.

Brevard Talent Group

Aspiring models on the east coast of central Florida are fortunate to have the expertise of Traci Danielli, president of the Brevard Talent Group. Traci has a thorough knowledge of the New York modeling industry and has connections with agents all over the world. She is part of a very successful mother-daughter team. Her mother, Lucy Heim, opened MDM Studios, Inc., in 1981. This is a licensed school in which the curriculum encompasses music, drama, and all areas of modeling. MDM is an excellent example of how a modeling school should be run, not only for its legitimacy but for the benefits it provides to all concerned. The school holds a "New Faces" Model Search annually (see page 225).

Agency address: Brevard Talent Group, 405 Palm Springs Boulevard, Indian Harbour Beach, FL 32937. Tel. (407) 773-1355. MDM Studios, Inc., address: 968 Pinetree Drive, Indian Harbour Beach, FL 32937. Tel. (407) 777-1344.

7
Canada

Canadian models are in demand all over the world. Canadian agents are held in high esteem by their international colleagues. Professionalism, friendliness, and a certain élan have combined to bring Canada into the world fashion spotlight. As I traveled through the fashion capitals, I was so impressed by the praise for this country and its models that I decided to explore the industry there.

Toronto is the major market and Montreal is next. Other cities such as Ottawa and Vancouver are growing markets, especially Vancouver, which is second only to Hollywood for filmmaking.

German-born Gaby Wagner, who owns the Zoom agency in Paris, told me: "I do most of my scouting in Canada. Every time I go there, I find star material. The models are fantastic! Models and agents are friendly and so professional."

The average earnings for a model are between $60,000 and $80,000 (Canadian). A new model can earn $30,000 (Canadian) and a top model $150,000 (Canadian). A foreign model with haute couture experience and correct working papers (obtained by the Canadian agency) can earn $60,000 (Canadian) in three months.

Toronto

In Toronto I interviewed Alecia Bell, who runs the family-owned International Top Models Agency, which was, coincidentally, the agency that had provided the models for an outstanding fashion show I had seen previously in this city. I asked her why Canadian models receive such rave reviews all over the world. She said: "Canada is a melting pot of ethnic backgrounds. We have communities of Ukrainians, Poles, and Scandinavians. Height, beautiful bone structure, wonderful hair and skin are in the genes." Alecia gave me her views on why the modeling industry has progressed so rapidly in the last few years: "We have several high-quality fashion magazines in Ontario. Our photographers are widely recognized in the international market. The trend is for photographers to apprentice in Europe. They bring their new skills back to Canada and become very competitive. In Toronto testing is comparable to, if not better than, Paris. Models can get fabulous tear sheets here. International agents go wild about our pictures."

International Top Models Agency

The agency, which opened in 1970, has a sister agency in Ottawa. One-fourth of the 125 models at the Toronto agency work in Osaka, Tokyo, Paris, Milan, Hamburg, and London. Models must be 5'9" and have good features. The 5'7" model must have a more commercial look for the local market. The men's division has thirty models. Its requirement is "a look that is in demand internationally."

This agency has fashion, print, and video divisions. Alecia's mother, Anne, is in charge of another agency, Butler, Rushton and Bell, which handles television, voice-over, dance, and theater.

Agency address: International Top Models Agency, 119 S. Padina Avenue, Suite 407, Toronto, Ontario M5V 2L1. Tel. (416) 979-9995. Fax (416) 979-8809.

Montreal

Folio Agence de Mannequin

In Montreal I spoke to Corinne Poracchia, a Frenchwoman who started the Folio Agence de Mannequin in 1985. Corinne was a model and stylist with an agency in Japan before moving to Montreal. She had this to say about the modeling profession in her city: "There is a lot of catalog work here. We have excellent photographers, which makes this a good place for a model to start a career. But this is a small market. A model with good potential must be prepared to travel. Foreign agents scout in Montreal and the opportunities for an international career are good."

Agency address: 295 De La Commune, Montreal, Quebec HZY 1E9. Tel. (514) 288-8080. Fax (514) 843-5597.

Vancouver

Agencies in Vancouver have a reputation for grooming models for Paris, Milan, and New York. Two such agencies are:

Charles Stuart Models and Actors, #214-1008 Homer St., Vancouver, B.C. V6B 2X1. Tel. (604) 683-2267. Fax (604) 683-2246. This is owned by Charles Stuart Quest.

VMH International Model and Talent Group, #200-1311 Howe Street, Vancouver, B.C. V6Z 1R7. Tel. (604) 687-4682. Fax (604) 669-3688. Agency has strong international modeling connections, and ties with the film industry.

8

International Modeling

International modeling can be a glamorous, exciting, fulfilling experience. It can also be a painful, lonely, devastating end to a dream. Hundreds of unqualified, unsupervised, hopelessly naive girls flock to Paris and Milan every year hoping to break into a modeling career. These are the girls who have major problems.

Before you attempt an international modeling career, you must have: a) the basic qualifications, b) a knowledgeable mother agent who knows the international market and deals with reputable international agents, c) maturity and emotional stability to cope with the demands of the profession, and d) a thorough awareness of what you are getting into.

Read this book thoroughly. I have traveled all over the world and interviewed the most experienced people in the business. If you know what to expect and are prepared, you will have overcome a major obstacle.

The agents who will establish your international career are the agents who are in the fashion capitals—New York, Chicago, Los Angeles, Dallas, Atlanta, Munich, Hamburg, Zurich, London, Paris, Milan, Madrid, Tokyo, and Sydney. These agents work together. Many agents in small towns and satellite markets do not know or understand the profession on this level. You must deal closely with an established agent in one of these major cities. Do not under any circumstances attempt to go to Europe under your own steam. It is imperative that you work through an agent in your native country. Write to the big agencies. Send them photographs and request an interview.

Why does a new model have to go to Europe? Europe is the finishing school of modeling, and agents have slightly more time to mold a career. There is also a greater concentration of magazines and fashion houses there than anywhere else in the world. This means greater opportunities to get tear sheets.

Here is some important advice. When you go to Europe do not expect to work right away. For the first six months do not measure success in terms of tear sheets and money—these will come in time. Remember that the experience of living and surviving in a foreign country is not only in itself a measure of success, it is also a powerful education. This is an outstanding opportunity to become a world traveler, learn languages, and study other cultures while learning the basic essentials of your profession. You will learn patience, how to cope with rejection, how to budget your finances, and how to smile and congratulate a friend who got a job instead of you, when inside you are crushed with disappointment and resentment. Until you learn all of this, you will never be a good model or have any hope of surviving in the profession.

Here is one encouraging fact: after many interviews worldwide, the one thing that impressed me was that the people at the top really care. The masterminds who own and run the world's top modeling agencies do care about their models, especially the newcomers. Some were models themselves. Some are parents. They too have experienced homesickness, success, rejection, fear, and doubt; but keep in mind that these people lead hectic lives and they certainly do not have time to babysit. A new generation of model agents is arriving on the scene. They are people who have spent years learning the business with big agencies in New York, Paris, or Milan and have now started out on their own. They have witnessed models' scarred egos and have learned from other agents' experiences and mistakes. Their agencies are small, allowing them time to be good at what they do and still have compassion for the newcomer. Some models do best with a small agency; others are less easily intimidated by the size of a large agency.

It is very important that you check the credentials of any agent with whom you deal. When television's *60 Minutes* exposed the alleged financial and sexual abuse of young models in Paris, the modeling world reeled from shock. Paris agents whose integrity was unquestionable were angered that their reputations might be tainted by the ugly publicity. When the furor subsided, however, it was agreed that the modeling profession would benefit from the publicity and Paris would be a safer place to work. Parents would pay more attention to their daughters' careers. Mother agents would check more closely the credentials of the foreign agents to whom they sent models, and models themselves would be more aware of what could happen in the business. Remember, there is no room for naivete in this profession. Don't be afraid to ask questions about your career. Your quest for knowledge will be respected.

The following information will keep you up to date on recent economic developments in Europe: The 1992 unification of Common Market countries (Belgium, Denmark, France, Germany, Greece, Italy, Ireland, Luxembourg, the Netherlands, Portugal, Spain, and the United Kingdom) saw a free-trade agreement among members of the European Economic Community (EEC). It enables Europeans to work in any member country they choose without working papers or permits. American models, however, still must adhere to immigration laws, which could become tighter. Although the agreement has made some smaller modeling agencies fear that big agencies will swallow them up, others feel that there will always be a need for small agencies and that the good ones will survive. Surely there are advantages and disadvantages to this change in Europe. But one thing is certain—the language barrier will remain unchanged!

Legal Aspects of International Modeling

Colin Claxon, an entertainment lawyer and co-owner of the Stars agency in San Francisco (see the chapter on legal matters), has this to say about the legal aspects of international modeling:

It is important for you to be aware of the differences in modeling internationally.

Your agent in the U.S., the "mother" agent, usually arranges to place you with an agency overseas—Paris, Milan, Tokyo, for example—and will receive a referral fee or percentage of the commission paid to the foreign agency. A good mother agency closely monitors your success overseas, as often as weekly. You should report all problems with your foreign agent to your mother agent. Never switch foreign agencies without first consulting your mother agency. All agencies differ and some may not be right for you, your look, or your career. If you do feel that a change is required, discuss it with your mother agency and let them make the arrangements. European agencies compete voraciously for models, and it is not uncommon for "runners" to hang around the front of agencies handing out cards and promising young models that they will make them stars. Avoid them. Before you leave the U.S., ask your mother agent to explain any foreign work restrictions to you.

Living expenses and a small allowance are usually advanced by European agencies, and some provide housing. It is not unusual for them to mark up their expenses above the actual cost. Some will collect full apartment rent from each model who shares an apartment, reaping a large profit. Don't stand for this. Find out the actual cost, complain, and report it to your mother agency.

Request an accounting of your expenses at least every month and verify your earnings. Never wait until you are leaving to attend to this. It always seems at such a time there is no one available to answer your questions.

Many European agencies will advance round-trip air-fare to Europe. An advance is a loan and will be deducted from your earnings.

If you make insufficient money to cover your expenses, the European agency will not expect you to reimburse them, if you have maintained your weight, have devoted sufficient time (usually two to three months), have worked hard and followed their instructions. You are a risk that they take, an investment, and if they fail to produce sufficient bookings to recover their costs, it is their loss. On the other hand, if you are discharged for misbehavior, if you change agencies, quit, or return home because of homesickness and the like, some agencies may attempt to recover their expenses by billing you, threatening legal action, or putting pressure on the mother agency.

Most foreign agencies properly deduct foreign income taxes, social security, and health taxes. Always get an explanation of these deductions.

Keep a copy of everything relating to your jobs: vouchers, tear sheets, and releases, etc. You may one day have to prove you didn't authorize use of a photo.

Now we will travel to the fashion capitals, explore the markets, and talk to the top agents in the business.

A final word of encouragement: American models are held in high esteem around the world for their professionalism, friendliness, and team spirit. Keep up the good work!

9

London

London is unique. Steeped in history and tradition, it is elegant, sophisticated, exciting, cosmopolitan, slightly eccentric, and enormous fun. It is a tough city for a model. Agents are selective and precise in what they want and expect. London has superb photographers and big business accounts. To keep pace with the high level of activity and degree of professionalism, agents prefer girls with experience. In Paris and Milan agents will make allowances for inexperience if a model has potential and will take the time to train her. This is not the case in London, where time means money. An inexperienced model will not work or make money quickly.

London agents are straightforward, honest, and efficient. They arrange work permits for foreigners and explain commissions and other financial details very clearly. I interviewed several agents in order to get a good overall picture of the London scene. The people to whom I spoke have been in the business for many years. While they differed on specific requirements, they all agreed on the need for a model to have money, insurance, grooming, personality, and to be well behaved. Their comments gave an excellent overall picture of the modeling scene in London.

One agent who has been in the business for over twenty

years was concerned with the number of American girls who arrive in Europe "on the flip of a coin." She said: "Agents in America tend to tell girls that if they go to Europe, they will work instantly. And school directors do not seem to have any control. They should take a tour and find out what is going on in Europe and Japan. American models should bring with them at least $2,000, medical insurance, and a return ticket. They must behave professionally at all times and have a lot of self-discipline."

The rules concerning modeling in the United Kingdom are laid down in a red book entitled *Terms, Conditions and Standards for the Engagement of Professional Models in Still Photography*. This is published jointly by the Association of Fashion, Advertising and Editorial Photographers, the Association of Model Agents, and the Institute of Practitioners in Advertising.

The Association of Model Agents establishes the integrity of its members.

Height requirements in London are 5'9" to 6'0" for women; 5'11" to 6'2" for men.

Elite Premier

The Premier Model Agency, which was in business at New Bond Street for seven years, has now merged with Elite in London and moved to larger premises in Covent Garden. Premier owners Carole White and Chris Owen, a brother-and-sister team who have extensive knowledge of the modeling profession, now run the new Elite Premier agency. Chris told me: "After several years of working together, the Elite people in London and Premier finally decided to merge. They have the benefit of our vast local experience in the London market, and we have the advantage of their top international models. This combination of a very high profile and large volume of work makes us the strongest agency in London." I asked Chris how he thought the economic unification of Europe would affect the modeling industry in England. "Everyone is looking to the whole of Europe now, not just the London market. It is not as parochial as it was five years ago. It is becoming more and more international. English and European models can move freely throughout the European Community and there has been a major breakthrough for American models. We can now obtain a full working visa for them within four weeks. The visa costs £150 for a year and is automatically renewable. This can only be done through the main modeling agencies in London. It is great news for the American model."

Elite Premier has a strong editorial image. The agency consists of the main, direct booking division of Elite; the Elite Premier division, which represents established English models, up-and-coming models, and brand-new faces; and a commercial division for television, video, and advertising campaigns. Runway models are also represented. Premier Photographic, which represents photographers, and Premier Men, which is under the direction of Sandra Sperka, continue to flourish at the new headquarters.

London is an excellent market for male models. The look for men is young and modern and models travel constantly to Paris, Milan, Germany, and Japan. Carole, who has been in the modeling business for over seventeen years and knows it well, had these comments on modeling as a career for men: "It is not a fleeting career. It can last a long time. Men don't take it quite as seriously as women. They use it as a tool to see the world. I think this is the right attitude. If a man does it for vain reasons, it puts people off. Clients don't like vain men."

I asked her for advice for new as well as experienced female models. She said: "They must be ambitious. A model must work with us on a fifty-fifty level. It takes as much effort on her part as ours. A girl should see modeling as an important career that will allow her to travel all over the world and make incredible amounts of money. But time is not on her side.

She must become professional very quickly, make money, and invest it well. She must think ahead. In five years it will be over.''

Carole told me that foreign girls obtain work quickly in London. "Clients know that a new face will only be in town for a short while and they want to see her." Her advice to potential models is: "Be confident! Take dancing and acting lessons. Learn how to move well. Know your look. I suggest that you save a few outfits you feel great in to wear to go-sees. Jeans are fine—with the right top, boots, and accessories. Take special care with your makeup. Even if you have a good book, you must be well turned out all the time. Clients are human. They want the girl in front of them to look as terrific as the girl in the book."

Chris is very active in the Association of Model Agents, which negotiates fees with clients on behalf of model agents. He said: "When we are negotiating, we have to keep in mind that a girl has about five years to make money and invest it. Once it is over, she is not likely to have the opportunity to make the same kind of money again. She doesn't know anything else, because she hasn't had the time to learn any other business. When agents receive complaints from clients that a model has been late for an appointment, we take disciplinary measures. But we have to remember that a model is not a tube of toothpaste or a can of beans. She is a human being who can make mistakes. We have to take all this into consideration when we are negotiating fees."

Agency address: Elite Premier, 40–42 Parker Street, London WC2B 5PH. Tel. 333 0888.

Select

Clare Castagnetti is one of four owners of Select, one of the most successful agencies in London. Clare feels that American models traveling to Europe for the first time should go to

London first in order to avoid a language barrier. "If girls are not secure, the culture shock will be overwhelming. Paris and Milan will really throw them if they are not prepared. It makes life so much simpler if they can understand the language. This business is tough enough as it is, and it is getting harder. Unless a girl is totally dedicated, she is wasting everyone's time. This is a very serious business."

Select represents girls as young as fourteen who work only during the school holidays, but prefers them to be sixteen or older. There are ninety models at this agency. Height for women is 5'9" to 6'0". For men, it is 6'0" to 6'2". The look at Select is the "young sophisticate." "The sort of girl seen in *Elle* and *Marie-Claire* magazines. We like models whose age cannot be determined."

Agency address: Select, 93 Newman Street, London, W1 P3LE. Tel. 631 4551. Fax 637-1301.

Take Two

This well-established agency is owned by Gabriella Palmano and Melissa Richardson. They take hundreds of telephone calls from would-be models every month, interview about eighty of these girls, and accept only one! Girls must be over 5'8" and under twenty-one years of age.

I talked at length with Gabriella Palmano. Here are her comments on a number of aspects of the business:

"There is a lot of hype on the street about how bitchy models are and how photographers want to get every girl into bed. But that is all it is—hype!

"A lot of girls don't realize what a strenuous and demanding career modeling is. Being photographed all day is hard work physically.

"It is important for a girl to know that personality is fifty percent of the business. It is as important as looks. If a girl is beautiful, and a pain in the neck to work with, she will be booked once and never again. A girl who is not as beautiful, but who is bright and has a pleasant personality, will be booked over and over again.

"A model always has to look her best—even if she has had a fight with her boyfriend and has been up all night crying. She can't come in here the next day looking and feeling a mess. A girl with a desk job might get away with it, but not a model. She must always be in top form."

Agency address: Take Two, 11 Garrick Street, London WC2R 9AR. Tel. 836 4501.

Models One Ltd.

With over twenty years in business, this is one of the few surviving original agencies in London. It has an excellent reputation.

The two owners, April Ducksbury and Jose Fonseca, are very selective when accepting girls from overseas. For accommodation purposes, they have an agency apartment and arrange for girls to live with families. "We make all of the arrangements when the girls come here, but we are very careful about whom we bring in." April told me: "We generally know who will work, but we can sometimes make a mistake. If a girl from the States doesn't work after three weeks, we call the mother agency, explain that her look isn't right for us, and arrange to send her to a market that will suit her better. If she is not up to our standards, or we think she is totally hopeless for Europe, we tell them this also. We are very truthful with the agencies.

"American agents should check all details very closely when they send girls to Europe. A number of agents do this, but many don't. It is very dangerous for a girl to just arrive in a foreign country. She wanders from agent to agent—even country to country—is not accepted, and then has to go back to America. I think this is terrible. If the proper arrangements have not been made, they haven't a chance of working. It is a waste of their time and it breaks their hearts. I feel so sad for them."

Models One does not pay air fare. The pay from clients in London is usually delayed for three months. Consequently, the agency will advance sixty percent of the invoice amount the first day a model works. Fifteen percent is kept in reserve in case there is a problem with clients concerning unprofessional behavior on the part of the model or to pay leftover bills from a model's doctor or dentist. The other twenty-five percent consists of the agency's twenty percent commission and a five percent fee for advancing money. April told me: "A model is better off financially in London than in Paris or Milan. In Milan, the agencies take fifty percent and the girls find it difficult to figure out just what they are earning, even if they are given a piece of paper with a lot of figures on it."

A good personality is strongly emphasized at this agency. Models must be professional, polite, well behaved, and easy to get along with. April told me: "Sometimes models behave very badly. We hate it when they start getting spoiled and stupid. If a model gets a reputation for being hard to work with we will ask her to leave. If there is the slightest inkling of drug use, they are out immediately. We don't want girls who are a bad influence on other models. Our reputation is at stake too. There are a lot of people involved and we are all in this together.

"American girls have incredible determination and their attitude toward becoming a model is the same as if they wanted to be a doctor or an accountant. However, we have found that when we have put them into a home to live with a family, they are very unhouse-trained, very undomesticated. An English girl is much quieter, much more considerate."

Models One Ltd. has a successful New Faces division for new models. This grooms new talent and develops careers. The fifteen- and sixteen-year-olds who are still at school are trained during school holidays. Minimum height for this agency is 5'8".

The men's division has thirty models and is very successful. "For our agency, a man has to look twenty-four or over and be 6′1″ to 6′4″. It is a very serious career for a male. If he is well groomed, charming, has a great personality, and gets on well with clients, he can work for a long time," said April.

Agency address: Models One Ltd., Omega House, 471–473 Kings Road, London SW10 OLU. Tel. 351 1195.

Storm

This Kensington agency was started by Sarah Doukas in July 1987. Sarah was a booker for over six years at the prestigious Laraine Ashton Agency in London before opening her own business. It was an immediate hit and is now one of the city's top agencies. Essential qualifications for girls are a height of 5′9″ or over, and a good personality. Sarah explained: "Our models have a specific look. We accept girls who will fit the *Elle* and *Vogue* market. But personality is very important. Even if a girl has all the physical attributes I might not take her if she doesn't have a good personality." Storm has a small number of fourteen- and fifteen-year-olds, but this age group is not encouraged. "We insist these young girls carry on with school and we keep in touch with them during the holidays."

The men's division was opened because male models in London wanted to work for Sarah as soon as they heard she had opened an agency. She accepted only a few at the beginning, but as work increased the division was permanently established. "We have two categories—the classic man, and the very interesting editorial man. Again personality is a top priority," said Sarah.

Agency address: Storm, 45 Marloes Road, London W8 6LA. Tel. 938 4033. Fax 937 8447.

General City Information

Other model agencies who are members of the Association of Model Agents:

Bookings, Studio 6, 27a Pembridge Villas, London W11 3EA. Tel. 221 2603.
Gavin's Models, 11 Old Burlington Street, London W1. Tel. 629 5231.
Profile, 15 Broad Court, off Drury Lane, London WC2B 5PH. Tel. 836 5282.
Planet, 47–48 New Bond Street, London W1Y 9HA. Tel. 409 7000. Fax 409 7070

Check telephone directory for other agencies.

Airports

There are two major airports serving London—Heathrow and Gatwick. When you arrive at either one you will clear Customs by a) following a red sign if you have goods to declare, or b) following a green sign if you do not. *Warning:* Do not make the wrong decision! Customs officials make regular spot checks in the green division.

Heathrow. The Underground (also called the Tube) connects this airport with all Tube stations in London, including the main British Rail stations. Service is excellent and the journey to the city center takes forty-five minutes. Cost is very reasonable. The Airbus, a double-decker red bus, goes into the city every ten minutes and takes about fifty minutes, rush hour traffic permitting. Plenty of room for luggage. There is also a green coach (bus) service called Flightline 767.

Gatwick. Thirty minutes from Victoria Station in the heart of London by the British Rail Gatwick Express. Trains run every fifteen minutes during the day and hourly at night. There is also the Flightline 777 coach service to Central London. All fares are very reasonable.

Transportation

Taxis. London is famous for its taxis. Fares are posted inside. Fare from Heathrow to the center of the city is roughly £20, depending on traffic. Drivers have a mind-boggling knowledge of the city. This is helpful for a model who is new in town, but taxis should not become habit-forming; they are expensive, and the Tube is often faster, espccially in rush hour. There is an extra charge for each piece of luggage or additional passengers.

Tube. This is the name given to the subway. You can buy one-way or round-trip tickets and daily, weekly, and monthly passes. Anything exceeding a daily pass requires a card bearing your photograph. This can be purchased at Victoria Station, and is a must for models. Tel. 222 1234 for twenty-four-hour travel information.

Buses. The best way to see London on your days off or when you have time is by the famous double-decker buses. Ticket conductors ride on the buses, and tickets are interchangeable with Tube tickets. They can also be bought separately.

There are a number of tours leaving from Piccadilly Circus. The best of these tours is the one that advertises "Original Tour of London." It takes about one hour forty-five minutes. The English are very orderly about lining up for buses. A bus will automatically stop at a compulsory red sign. If, however, a bus stop sign has REQUEST written on it, put out your hand to stop the bus.

Cars. Beware! Cars drive on the left side of the road. Look to the *right* before crossing.

Currency

The pound sterling is the monetary unit. The symbol is £ and it is made up of 100 pence, referred to as "p." Money comes in bank notes and coins. Check these closely until you are used to the currency.

Banks

You get the best rate of exchange at a bank. Every major bank has branches all over London. Hours are 9:30 A.M.–3:30 P.M. Mon.–Fri.; off-hour service is available at the airports.

Telephone

Models live on the telephone! The tall red telephone booths are called kiosks.

City code for London is 71, but drop this when dialing within the city. To call an international operator, dial 155.

For local calls, the new phones are easy to use. If you have a number of calls to make, you can deposit a coin and the amount you have used will appear on a small screen. However, if you do have to use one of the old telephones, a little explanation will be useful. (I still find them nerve-racking!) Dial the number first, and then as soon as the party at the other end answers (an English person will either say "Hello" or is more likely to say his own telephone number) you will hear a series of fast pips. You will think you have been cut off, but you have not. Quickly deposit the required coins (the amount will be posted) and be sure to give them quite a push to make them go through the slot. The connection has now been made. Another series of horrid pips will sound when more money has to be inserted. I warn you this system is ghastly!

To make a direct call to the United States, dial 010 + 1 + area code + number. Parents or friends calling London from the U.S. dial 011 + 44 + 71 + number for a direct call. The international access code is 011; 44 is the country code; 71 is the city code for London, 81 for outer London.

A collect call is called a "reverse charge" call and can only be made from a private phone. If you don't have a private phone, you can go to the Westminster International Telephone Bureau, 1 Broadway, SW1, make a direct call, and pay at the end of it. Hours are 9:00 A.M.–5:30 P.M. including weekends. This can also be done at the Trafalgar Square post office, and at both airports at special telephone offices.

In an emergency situation, dial 999.

Postal Service

Main post office: 24–28 William IV Street, WC2N 4DL. Tel. 239 2000. Open twenty-four hours seven days. Regular post office hours are Mon.–Fri. 9:00 A.M.–5:30 P.M. (sometimes 6:00 P.M.).

American Express

Central office is located at 6 Haymarket, London SW1. Tel. 930 4411.

Tourist Information

London Tourist Board, 26 Grosvenor (pronounced "Grovenor") Gardens, London SW1. Tel. 730 0791.

Embassies/Consulates

Canada: Canada House, Trafalgar Square, London SW1. Tel. 629 9492.
USA: 24 Grosvenor Square, London W1. Tel. 499 900.

Toilet

Do not refer to a toilet as a bathroom. People will look at you in amazement. I heard one snooty hotel doorman ask an American gentlemen who inquired as to the whereabouts of the bathroom: "Does sir wish to take a bath?" This facility is called a lavatory or toilet. Signs outside read W.C., LADIES, or GENTLEMEN.

Time Difference

London is on Greenwich Mean Time, except during May through October when clocks are moved ahead one hour to establish British Summer Time. GMT is five hours ahead of Eastern Standard Time in the United States.

Water

Water can be drunk from the tap all over England except for the possible exception of trains, where signs will indicate otherwise.

Electric Current

220 to 240 volts, AC. You will need a converter unless you have dual voltage equipment, and an adaptor for British sockets. These can be bought at major department stores or electrical shops.

Recommended Street Map

Agencies recommend the "A–Z," which includes a Tube map.

Language

English. For the benefit of American models, here is a list of words that have different meanings:

AMERICAN	BRITISH
pantyhose	tights
raincoat	mac
dieting	slimming
bathroom (meaning toilet)	toilet, lavatory (you will see W.C. signs posted also)
apartment	flat
umbrella	brolly
flat (as in tire)	puncture
shot (medical)	injection
drugstore	chemist or pharmacy
elevator	lift
sidewalk	pavement (American friends thought I was weird when I told my children to play on the pavement)
trunk (of a car)	boot
hood (of a car)	bonnet
cookies	biscuits (models must never eat them!)
candy	sweets (nor these!)
check (restaurant)	bill
gasoline	petrol
truck	lorry

Note also that in Britain, when the date is written, the day comes first and then the month, e.g., 2/1/95 is January 2, 1995. In the United States it would be written 1/2/95.

Police Emergency

Telephone 999. No money is required. The same applies when you dial "0" for operator assistance.

10

Germany

Germany is the biggest fashion exporter in the world. Hamburg and Munich are major markets and have a high concentration of catalog work. Once established, a model can earn reasonable money, pay expenses, and live well. However, this is not really the country for tear sheets. Most of these will be unsuitable for portfolios in Milan or Paris. This can be frustrating, but the situation is improving. You should also know that television commercials are extremely limited. Therefore you cannot rely on this medium to supplement your income to any great extent. There is a big market in Germany for male models.

Germany runs on rules. It runs efficiently, to the benefit of everyone. So do the agencies. Obey the rules and you will be successful. Break them, or try to bend them, and you could be sent home.

There is a finance company behind every agency. The agency handles the model and represents him or her to clients. The finance company backs the model financially and handles commissions received for administration and organization. When a model lists with a German agency, working permission is granted automatically. She does not pay tax on what she earns. (This is paid to her country of residence.) She works for a fee, pays a commission to the finance company, and the rest is hers. This situation is unique to Germany. Male and female foreign models are in great demand here.

A German girl is expected to finish high school and university, or an apprenticeship to a trade. Parents insist on this. As a result, there are few German models. By the time they have finished their education it is too late to start. It is unheard of for a girl to take a year off from her studies to model and then return to school. And as a general rule German men don't model. Hence the demand for foreigners.

The two major cities in which models work are Hamburg and Munich. There are excellent agencies in both cities. Let us take a look at each city.

Hamburg

This is an ideal place for a young model to start in the profession on an international level. Parents can relax and breathe a sigh of relief if their son or daughter signs with an agency here. It is very safe, low key, conservative, and sophisticated. The people are friendly and most of them speak English. There are no muggings and few robberies—a portfolio left in a restaurant will be there two days later. People in the profession are honest. A deal is a deal. The look here is young, fresh, girl-next-door.

Two highly respected personalities who owned their own model agencies in Hamburg for many years had strong comments and words of advice for new models arriving in this city. Sebastian Sed, who invented the Sed Card—the composite that is a model's indispensable work tool—stressed the need for models to obtain health insurance before leaving home.

Asked about the problems confronting new, young models, he told me: "They have the very wrong idea that once they have arrived here everything is going to be easy. They expect too much. They think this is a sure road to success and they are going to be stars. This is probably the fault of the people who run the modeling schools."

I asked Sebastian how long it takes a girl to start to work. He explained: "The commercial model who is tall, has a good smile, beautiful hair, and the right look can work after ten days. She will always be right for catalog and she can also do editorial work. The editorial girl who is more extraordinary, more exotic but not necessarily beautiful, tends to be more successful—eventually. She can take six to nine months to get going. That's the hard part. And of course, some don't make it at all."

Eileen Green is well known and admired in international modeling circles. She has all the charm and humor of the Irish and a beautiful brogue to match. She has a wealth of knowledge of the history of the business and the people who founded and developed it. Eileen gave me her views on modeling schools. "Students should be told to respect the country they go to and to learn something about it. Europe is a great learning experience."

Eileen is concerned about girls who arrive in Hamburg overweight and try to solve the problem by crash dieting. She sees this as a great danger. She told me: "It is better for a girl to stay at home and lose the weight. It is very frustrating for a model to lose a job because she is too heavy. She must be honest about her measurements. Clothes are made to a certain size, and it is terribly sad when a client wants to book a girl who has a super look and then finds out that she is one or two sizes larger than the size she has printed on her card. It is awful if this results in her being sent home from a trip at her own expense."

On the subject of rejection, Eileen said: "There are so many reasons why a model might not be booked. She must never take it personally and become depressed." On the model-agent relationship her advice is: "A modeling agent offers a service to a model for a fee. The combination of model and agent must be good. Both must be happy. I advise any young model to shop around and if she is not happy, to change agents. The agent also has the privilege of asking her to leave."

Eileen advises young girls who have never had to live on a budget to ask questions about rent, transportation, and food and to forget about buying clothes until they are working and covering expenses. She emphasizes that models from overseas must have travel and health insurance and, as a further security measure, enough money to support themselves for at least a couple of months. Money should always be in the form of travelers checks. "Modeling is a gamble. These young people are not walking into security," she said.

Model Team

Mention the Model Team agency to anyone in the business and it is acknowledged with admiration and respect. It is owned by Sonja ("Soni") and Ralf Ekvall, a Swedish couple who opened the agency eighteen years ago, making it the oldest model agency in Hamburg. It is large, with 400 models on the books; half of the 250 girls are American. The 150-strong male division is also very successful. Soni works closely with the Ford agency in New York and has judged the "Face of the Eighties" contest, a glossy production organized by the Ford agency, now called "Super Model of the World."

Soni is tall, striking, and elegant, with a keen eye for talent. Her judgment is seldom wrong. A beautiful suite of offices provides a glamorous and functional setting for her efficient, friendly staff. Soni scouts internationally. Girls must be 5′9″ to 6′0″ tall, have long legs, "be skinny enough," have excellent hair and skin and a good smile. A little variation is allowed on the perfect 34-24-34 body statistic. Girls who have slight measurement problems are told to swim and work out in a gym. Men are warned about playing too many sports or doing too much bodybuilding; musclebound legs and very broad shoulders are a no-no. Soni explained: "There is a great deal of fashion here, a great deal of catalog work, but models have to be able to fit into the clothes."

Asked about her keen sense of judgment in selecting models, she said: "When I see a girl I can tell instinctively if she is good. The way she presents herself to me is the way she will eventually present herself to a client. Of course, even when I am convinced, I can be wrong. A girl might be very homesick and very unhappy, and if this is the case, she will not present a positive image to the client. If a girl does not do well and I have to send her home, she does not have to repay her fare. I consider that my investment—a business investment. It is very, very unusual that a girl doesn't work at all because I am so picky when I make my original selection."

When a new girl arrives at Model Team, a lot of time is spent teaching her the agency's policy, how the modeling business works, and about Hamburg itself. Soni told me: "I was a foreigner here once. I know it can be frightening for a young girl. A good agent will tell her models that she believes in them and make them feel happy and confident. A lot of success lies in planning. When I know a foreign girl is coming, I ring up good photographers, good hairdressers, and get clothes for tests. I treat it as if the girl were on the job." She added: "If a girl arrives with a good book she can work within a few days. If it has to be changed, it will take her two weeks. There are a lot of good magazines here. It is a very big market." Specifically, Soni stresses the need for a model to obtain health insurance prior to leaving home.

Agency address: Model Team, Schleuterstrasse 60, 20146 Hamburg 13. Tel. 414 10 30.

Body and Soul

Pia Kohles who heads this agency has a wealth of experience in both the advertising and model agency business. She is also a booker and a scout. Explaining the advantage of wearing these various hats, she said: "At every agency the bookers know what type of model clients want because they have direct contact with them. Scouts don't work with the clients. They travel, find cute girls who don't necessarily work, and the whole thing becomes a disaster. In my case, I scout girls around the world knowing what clients are looking for, and when I get back to the booking table I know who is coming to the agency. I have met the girl. She arrives within two months and she works. I have never had a problem. Very occasionally I have brought a girl to Hamburg having only seen her book. Then I have found that she looks different in person. We are disappointed. Things don't go well. The girl is disappointed and the mother agent is too. Again it is a disaster."

Discussing the problem of teenagers arriving in Europe in pursuit of a modeling career, Pia told me: "Every year hundreds of girls from America and Canada go to Milan during their summer break. They sit there with three pictures in their books and it is a waste of time. Eighty percent of these girls don't have a chance in Milan. It would be much better if they came to a smaller agency in Hamburg where there is a lot of constant work in catalog, beauty, body, and hair. Agents will advise them to go to Portugal or Greece to work on their books and then come back to Hamburg for more experience. Then they can go to Milan and Paris.

"When new girls arrive at Body and Soul, they have an in-depth discussion with a staff member during which they learn about the agency and the city. They are accommodated with a Hamburg family. Everything possible is done to launch a successful career."

The agency only represents women. There are about 250 models aged between sixteen and thirty. Minimum height requirement is 5'9".

Agency address: Body and Soul, Heinrich Barth Str. 21, 2146 Hamburg. Tel. 41 20 91. Fax 41 04 748.

The following information is typical of the type of information given to models by agencies all over the world. It gives insight into how an agency operates and what is expected of a model.

Hamburg Hints

1. Full-day Booking — Nine hours including lunch.
2. Half-day Booking — Four hours, approximately.
3. Overtime — The first half-hour is "give & take" and thereafter each hour is chargeable. *Agency must be informed within 24 hours* of the booking for overtime to be negotiated. *Please make a note of agency booker.*
4. Expenses — Trips outside of Germany, clients usually pay most expenses including hotel/lunch, etc. Flight bookings within Germany, client pays hotel and breakfast only, plus any taxi expenses incurred *in the city or town of work*.

    Taxi expenses in Hamburg to the airport are not chargeable. Expenses are paid only if all hotel and taxi bills are received by the agency *within 5 days of booking completion*.
5. Traveling Time — Catalogs do not pay traveling time if the booking is for five days or more. Editorial or advertising trips are negotiable re traveling time.
6. Cancellation — For single-day booking, models must cancel minimum 48 hours before day of booking. For more than single-day bookings, models

must cancel equivalent to the length of the booking (*i.e., with a five-day booking the model must cancel at least five days before*).

7. Accessories — Girls are expected to arrive at all bookings fully made up, *with clean hair*, and with bodystockings, etc. Any other accessories will be given as an extra with booking details.

8. Go-sees — Go-sees are generally arranged in the mornings in the Agency, never over the phone.

9. Cash from Agency — Generally Thursday & Friday afternoons only, between noon and 3 P.M.; for special arrangements phone agency.

10. Cash from Client — If cash is paid by client for fee/flight, etc., a full breakdown of the total amount must be given to the agency *within 24 hours*.

11. Next-day Bookings — Agency must be phoned before 5:30 P.M. (17:30).

12. Trips Abroad — Models are responsible for visas (phone your consulate), passport, and vaccinations.

Beware: — Any model not showing for a booking is liable for the day's full production cost, including other models' fees.

Not showing for a trip also includes liability for all flight, travel, and hotel costs plus fees incurred by client, photographer, stylist, other models, etc.

The model will be sued in country

of residence or the costs deducted
from model's account.

Any model late for booking loses
not only the hourly rate for the
late time, but also must pay other
models' waiting time.

General City Information

Airport (Flughafen)

Hamburg's airport, Fuhlsbüttel, is linked to the city center
by taxi or a combination of bus and subway. You will find
the bus stop to the left of the exit doors on the lower level of
the airport. The Airport Express bus leaves every ten minutes
for the Ohlsdorf station, which is serviced by the U-Bahn and
S-Bahn trains. A train for the desired destination can be taken
from here.

Transportation

Taxis. Fare begins at 3 deutsche marks (DM). If you call a
taxi by phone, the meter will start at DM4. It is not considered correct behavior to hail a taxi from the side of the road.
One must find a taxi stand.

U-Bahn. This is the name given to the underground or subway
system. Tickets for the rapid-transit trains, serving the Underground and S-Bahn local lines, are also valid on buses and passenger ferries. U-Bahn tickets can be purchased on a single or
daily basis at any station. A weekly or monthly pass, which
requires a photo card, can be bought at the Hauptbahnhof,
which is the central station. The last two are not recommended
by agents for models who plan only a short stay in Hamburg,
or who travel constantly, back and forth, to other countries.

I am going to outline the procedure for buying a single
U-Bahn ticket, because on my first day in Hamburg, I trav-

eled all over the city without one. I just did not know how or where to buy it, and I could not find an official to ask. Here is a step-by-step description: At the station there is a board with a list of numbers next to a board with a list of destinations. Find your planned destination and press the corresponding button. The cost of the journey will be shown and you can insert the correct amount. Paper money is not accepted. A daily ticket is represented by a button with a *T* on it. Press the button; the ticket price will appear and you can insert the correct amount.

Buses. Tickets may be purchased from the driver and they are interchangeable with daily U-Bahn tickets.

Cars. Vehicles drive on the right side of the road.

Currency

The deutsche mark (DM) is the unit of currency. One deutsche mark equals 100 pfennigs, or DM1 – 100 pfg.

Banks

Mon., Tues., Wed., and Fri. 9:00 A.M.–1:00 P.M. and 2:30 P.M.–4:00 P.M.
Thurs. 9:00 A.M.–1:00 P.M. and 2:30 P.M.–6:00 P.M.
Closed on weekends.

Telephone

Making a telephone call can be a challenge in foreign cities. In Hamburg, I met a couple of models who, every morning, in order to check in with their agency, had to get up, dress, walk (usually in the rain) several blocks to the nearest telephone box and, clutching the correct change, stand in line to check in for the day! There are locks on many apartment phones and models may only receive incoming calls.

Long Distance. It is possible to dial direct; e.g., for the United States dial 00 + 1 + area code + number. A collect call can be made only from a private phone or at the main post office. Dial 0010 and you will hear a voice say: *"Bitte warten Sie,"* which means "Please wait." When you hear the next voice, ask for an international operator. Long-distance calls can be made from the Hauptbahnhof.

Specially marked phone booths will enable you to make international calls, but you will need to have a great deal of change. Also, phones that have their numbers clearly printed on the outside can be used to receive calls.

Parents or friends wishing to call Hamburg would dial 011 + 49 + 40 + number. The international access code is 011; country code for Germany is 49; city code for Hamburg is 40.

Postal Service

The post office in the Hauptbahnhof central station is open twenty-four hours. Other post office hours are: 8:00 A.M.-3:30 P.M.

American Express Office

This office is located at Rathausmarkt 5. Tel. 33 11 41.

Embassies/Consulates

Canada: Esplanade 41–47. Tel. 35 18 05.
U.S.A.: Alsterufer 27. Tel. 44 10 61.

Toilet

HERREN (men), DAMEN (women).

Time Difference

Hamburg is one hour ahead of Greenwich Mean Time (GMT), six hours ahead of Eastern Standard Time (EST), and nine hours ahead of Pacific Standard Time. Daylight Saving Time is in effect between April and September.

Tipping

Service is included. If service is outstanding, a small additional gratuity is appropriate. Porters: DM2 per bag. This is a good tip for any service.

Water

Water is safe to drink except on trains.

Electric Current

220 volts, AC.

Recommended Street Map

The Falk Plan.

Police Emergency

Telephone 110.

Munich

Munich is the capital of Bavaria, the beer capital of the world, and the fashion capital of Germany. The German name is München, which means Place of the Monks. The Münchners are hard, dedicated workers who make a point of taking time out to enjoy life. Oktoberfest, the beer-drinking festival, and Fasching, a carnival that lasts from the Epiphany on January 6 to Mardi Gras or Shrove Tuesday, are world-famous festivities that draw crowds from all over the world. Models, designers, photographers, makeup artists, and stylists crowd into Munich during Mode Woche—Fashion Week—which takes place in March and October.

Life is pleasant, easygoing, and safe, and considerably less formal than in Hamburg. Models love this city, but they have to be really good at their profession in order to work here. The situation in the business has changed in the last few years. At one time, for example, it was considered chic to book an American model because it was a different thing to do. This is not the case anymore unless the model is very good. Clients are not eager to work with beginners. They will pay high booking fees, but they insist on value for money, and that means experience. It is definitely not easy to get tear sheets here. And the idea that a new model can make money quickly is totally wrong. One booker took time out from a busy schedule to have coffee with me and give me some insight into the business. She emphasized the disillusionment young models face when they arrive in Munich as a result of misleading information given to them before leaving home. "It is very wrong of agents in other countries to tell girls that if they come to Germany they will make enough money to go to Paris and Milan to get tear sheets. This idea is very wrong. The fact is, you need tear sheets to do *catalog* work here."

The height requirements are a minimum of 5'8" for a girl—although as every agent will tell you anywhere in the world, there is always the exception to this rule. Sometimes a girl who is 5'7" and in some way absolutely outstanding will work constantly. But I do emphasize that this is not usual. A male model must be 6'1" or a little taller. In Germany and Switzerland, models are expected to bring their own makeup to jobs and know how to apply it well. They are also expected to have their own accessories.

A model does not need a fabulous book but it must be good and show that she has experience. She must be easy to work with. Clients will not tolerate arrogance or lack of profession-alism. In fact they will happily pass over a beautiful girl for one less pretty with a great personality. Time is money. They want to get the job done quickly and well and enjoy doing it at the same time.

Nova Models

I had the pleasure of interviewing, at length, Ingrid Reiling, a striking blonde and a truly gracious lady who owns and runs the Nova Models agency with her husband, Norman. She was very concerned about the misconception with which new girls arrive in Munich. "Girls are told by agents that they can come here to do catalog work without having a book. This is just not so. It is very difficult. A couple of years ago clients would call us and ask us to send over a few girls. Now they ask to see a card first and then, if they are interested, they will ask to see the girl and her book. If the book isn't good enough they won't book her."

Modeling is extremely competitive in Munich. Clients are always looking for new faces, and they can choose from models who flock into the city from all over Europe and America. There really are many beautiful German girls and their sense of fashion is innate. But amazingly enough, they look down on modeling as a profession. It doesn't have the same prestige for them. Ingrid explained: "The term *model* has a different connotation here. If a girl says she is a model anywhere else in the world, everyone thinks it's fantastic. It is every girl's dream. But here I have to convince a girl to become a model. I have to bring her to the agency and prove to her that we are professional and that she can be serious about her work."

We talked about how the business has changed in the past few years. "At one time a girl had to be beautiful. Now all kinds of looks are in—even ugly! It is very strange for an agent to see a girl who she thinks is ugly but who she feels has a chance."

Klages Models has merged with Nova and the agency represents women and men. Minimum age and height requirement for women is sixteen and 5'9"; age range for men is twenty to forty and the minimum height requirement is 6'0". Commenting on male modeling in Munich, men's booker Sylvia Graef said: "It is always more difficult for men. There are so many on the market and only a few good ones. Clients don't use a lot of male models. There is great competition for work."

Agency address: Nova Models, Antonionstrasse 3, 8000 Munich 40. Tel. 89 34 70 73.

Heide Themlitz Talents, Models

This Munich agency has been in existence since the early seventies. The license was taken over by Heide Themlitz in May 1982. Heide is soft-spoken, extremely charming, and highly respected by her peers on the international circuit. She is very concerned about the situation facing new models arriving in Europe. She has German models, girls from other parts of Europe, and American models. Heide explained that the Americans have the toughest time for a number of reasons. Europeans are used to traveling from country to country and dealing with different cultures and languages. Americans are not. Also European models know that in Germany and Switzerland they are required to carry accessories with them at all times, and also makeup, which they must know how to apply expertly. Americans generally are not aware of this when they arrive.

These points are very important in this country. Another major point that Europeans seem to be more aware of is the need to have money in order to survive until they work. Heide told me: "American agents should prepare girls for Europe. They send them to Milan, where they can't possibly work without good books. They don't have money, become depressed, and gain weight. They sit around and nobody cares for them. American girls are pushed into the profession at a very early age. They don't know how to handle it and many of them don't know how to behave properly. We always have problems when we rent them an apartment. We have problems with their telephone bills. And they don't have much respect for other people's possessions. They do not receive good advice from their agents in America.

"When I accept a girl at my agency I consider her my responsibility. If she arrives without money I will give her some. Even if I never get it back I consider that was my responsibility. Models must *never* arrive in Europe without money. That is why they become involved in the drug scene."

Agency address: Internationale Talents Modelle, Ohmstrasse 5, 8000 Munich 40. Tel. 397 018.

Summing up, then, we can say that Germany is the best place to break into the international modeling scene provided you have enough money for accommodation, food, and tests for a few months. If you do not have a reasonable book or reasonable pictures, you must be prepared to be very patient until you get them. Be pleasant, courteous, and respect the people and their culture. If you do this you will have a terrific experience, learn the business from experts, and be on your way to success.

General City Information

Airport (Flughafen)

Flughafen Riem is about six miles from the center of the city. Buses leave from the Arrivals building every twenty minutes for the Hauptbahnhof, the main train station, in the city center.

111

Transportation

Taxis. Start at DM3 and can be hailed in the street or found at a taxi stand.

U-Bahn. (See page 105.)

Buses. Excellent bus system with tickets interchangeable with trams and U-Bahn.

Cars. Vehicles drive on the right side of the road.

Currency

The deutsche mark is the unit of currency. One deutsche mark equals 100 pfennigs, or DM1 = 100 pfg.

Banks

Mon.–Fri. 8:30 A.M.–12:30 P.M. or 1:00 P.M., and 1:30 P.M. or 2:30 P.M.–4:00 P.M.
Tuesdays open until 5:30 P.M. or 6:00 P.M.

Telephone

(See the information on p. 106.) The city code for Munich is 89. To make a direct international call, dial the access code for the country you are in, the country code for the country you are calling, the city code and then the number. For example, to call Munich from the United States, dial 011 (international access code in the U.S.), 49 (country code for Germany), 89 (city code for Munich), and then the number of the party. To direct-dial the U.S. from Munich, dial 010 for the operator and then ask for the international operator. This must be done from a private telephone or the main post office.

Postal Service

Main post office is at the Hauptbahnhof central station and is open twenty-four hours. Other post office hours are: Mon.-Fri. 8:00 A.M.-3:30 P.M., Sat. 8:00 A.M.-noon. Always make sure that you have the correct postage for airmail.

American Express Office

Location is: Reiseburo 2, Promenadplatz 6. Tel. 21 99 0.

Embassies/Consulates

Canada: Max-Joseph-strasse 6. Tel. 55 85 31.
U.S.A.: Königinstrasse 5–7. Tel. 23 01 1.

Toilet

Look for the signs: HERREN (men), DAMEN (women), or W.C.

Time Difference

(Same as Hamburg and the rest of Germany)

Electric Current

220 volts, AC.

Recommended Street Map

The Falk Plan, which can be purchased at any department store.

Police Emergency

Telephone 110.

11

Zurich

Zurich is the fashion capital of Switzerland. It is also the country's largest city and banking center. It has tremendous Old World charm and is truly delightful. Life is conservative and the Zurichers are organized and to the point. Sometimes their efficient, businesslike manner is mistaken for arrogance and coldness. This is not the case. They are extremely courteous and helpful. You, in turn, must be polite, punctual, and professional.

This is probably the best city in Europe for an experienced model to make excellent money. A beginner, however, will not do well. There are few photographers for testing, and a model must have a strong book and tear sheets to prove that she is experienced. There is very little editorial work. Television advertising is minimal and poorly paid. This is the city for catalog and commercial work.

Here is an important point: models must have their own accessories and makeup and know how to apply it well. This is imperative for catalog work.

Official papers are essential for living and working in Switzerland. Everyone pays taxes. Agency fees range from 25 to 30 percent and include commission, accident and health insurance, and the 8 percent government tax.

Zurich has a serious drug problem. Imprisonment and/or deportation are the penalties. Agencies will not tolerate the slightest sign of drug use.

There are no underground trains, and taxis are expensive. It is wise to learn the bus and tram systems quickly. The service is excellent, easy, and inexpensive.

Switzerland is bordered by France, Italy, and Germany. The look that is "in" for these countries is "in" for Zurich about two months later. Foreign models are in demand. Swiss men do not model, which makes Zurich a great city for male models. American men are very popular. However, the Swiss do not consider modeling a "proper" profession for a girl. She is expected to finish school and university, by which time it is too late to start a modeling career.

Françoise Rubartelli was first a model, and then an agent for many years in Zurich. She is now retired and living in Italy. Françoise laughed when she recalled her decision to become a model despite protests to her parents from relatives and friends. "My parents were asked: 'Your daughter is from a good family. Does she really need to do this?' " Her career decision was definitely frowned upon.

I interviewed Françoise while she was an agent. Her concern was that models are getting younger and younger. She told me: "In Milan, I have seen fourteen- and fifteen-year-olds sitting on staircases drinking milk. They were not working, couldn't speak the language, and were so lonely and unhappy. I blame the parents for this terrible situation."

We discussed the problems facing models trying to start out in the business in Zurich. Françoise explained: "It is very difficult for a beginner. Sometimes I see a girl and I know that she will be good. But when I tell a client this and ask them to give her a chance, they refuse. Then I have to send her to Italy for tear sheets. She has to start somewhere, but it can't be Zurich. A good book and tear sheets are essential. At one time we were flooded with fifteen- and sixteen-year-olds who had good portfolios because they worked with a good photographer in America. But they came here without accessories or makeup and hadn't a clue about how to handle themselves. The clients were angry. A model is not usually booked from her book, but if she is, she had better be good. When Swiss people get mad, they get mad, and they don't forget!''

Time Model Management

Time Model Management (founded by Françoise Rubartelli) is the oldest agency in Switzerland. It is located in the old part of the city. The streets are cobbled and the area so quaint. Judy Stäuble and Lisa Giger are the owners. Judy told me: "This is a pure money market. It is catalog and advertising work, not editorial work. Here models start in their teens—by their mid-twenties their careers are more or less over. A man's career lasts longer. My advice to young people starting in the business is to be very careful and to listen to different people before they make a career decision."

Height requirements at this agency are 5'9" to 5'11" for women and 6'0" for men.

Agency address: Time Model Management, Spitalgasse 4, 8001 Zurich. Tel. 261 60 40.

PMS (Photo Model Service)

The same height requirements and conditions hold true at PMS, which is owned by Marianne Fischer. Marianne has an intense knowledge of the modeling business. She was exceedingly gracious and eager to offer advice and information to help a model feel at home in Zurich and work as much as possible. She also emphasized the need for a strong book and tear sheets and sends models to Milan for tear sheets if necessary. Marianne explained: "Switzerland is the best place, moneywise, for a girl who is experienced. We pay our models on the same day that they work—we are the only agency in Europe that does this. Zurich is small and models soon get to know each other, so there is no problem with homesickness. There is a lot of work here and time passes quickly."

There are about twenty-five to thirty girls at this agency. If a girl is experienced, she can arrive in Zurich with about $300. If she has not worked within a month, she is advised to relocate.

Agency address: PMS, Rieterstrasse 21, 8002 Zurich. Tel. 202 37 44.

General City Information

Airport

Zurich Airport is about seven miles from the center of the city. There are taxi, bus, and train services and the journey takes about ten minutes.

Transportation

Taxis. These are expensive and models are advised not to use them. A service charge is included in the fare. For taxi service, call Taxi-Zentrale, Tel. 44 44 41.

Underground. There is no underground system.

Buses and Trams. This system is cheap, efficient, and easy to learn. To buy a ticket, find a vending machine and find your destination, which will be in the red, yellow, or blue areas displayed on the machine. Press the appropriate button and the fare will light up in red. Insert the correct number of coins. Single or daily tickets can be bought at each stop.

Weekly and monthly tickets are not advisable for models who are planning a short stay. They take the form of a photo card, which is obtained at the Central Train Station. Anyone found traveling without a ticket will be fined on the spot.

Cars. Traffic drives on the right side of the road.

Currency

The unit of currency is the Swiss franc (SF or F). One Swiss franc equals 100 rappen. Money can be changed at banks, travel offices, the airport, and Central Station (6:20 A.M.-11:30 P.M. daily).

Banks

Hours are 8:15 A.M.-4:30 P.M.

Telephone

To call collect, dial 111 for local operator; 191 for international. For direct calls to the United States, dial: 00 + 1 + area code + number of party. Parents and friends wishing to call Zurich from the U.S. dial: 011 + 41 + 1 + number. You cannot dial overseas from a pay phone. This must be done at a post office. Make the call and pay at the counter afterward.

Postal Service

The main post office is Sihlpost. Hours are: Mon.-Fri. 7:30 A.M.-6:30 P.M. Sat. 7:30 A.M.-11:00 A.M. Sun. closed. All other post offices close for lunch. There are special evening, weekend, and emergency hours at the Sihlpost and at the Central Station post office.

American Express

Office is located at Bahnhofstrasse 20. Tel. 211 83 70.

Embassies/Consulates

Canada: P.O. Box 3000, Berne 6. Tel. (31) 44 63 81.
U.S.A.: Zollikerstrasse 141. Tel. 55 25 66.

Toilet

DAMEN (Ladies); HERREN (Men) or MÄNNER; TOILETTEN; or
W.C.

Time Difference

Zurich is one hour ahead of Greenwich Mean Time (GMT)
and six hours ahead of Eastern Standard Time (EST). It has
adopted Daylight Saving Time.

Electric Current

220 volts, AC.

Recommended Street Map

Offizieller Stadtplan Zürich und Umgebung. This map includes the bus and tram routes.

Police Emergency

Dial 117.

12

Paris

Paris is chic, exciting, and romantic. Love and fashion are its greatest exports. The Parisians have a passion for life and enjoy their leisure time with as much Gallic gusto as they do their work. The older generation is deliciously arrogant on the surface, but gracious, charming, and extremely receptive once introductions have been made. The young do not have this aloof veneer and are easily approachable. And, as is always the case with the young, they make friends easily with their contemporaries.

Paris fashion has had a dynamic impact on the world, thanks to the creative genius of Dior, St. Laurent, Chanel, Courrèges, and many others. Frenchwomen are brilliant at accessorizing, but they would look chic in a sheet and Wellington boots. A young model can learn a lot by looking at the store windows on the Champs-Elysées or sitting in a sidewalk café watching the parade of fashion go by.

An organization known as Le Syndicat des Agences De Mannequin (S.A.M.) gives the guidelines to agencies for rates, rules, and regulations, and defines the laws on royalties, television, and poster rates.

Certain documents are required in order to live and work in France. It is mandatory that you have these and that they be kept up to date. You will hear the words "social security," or "*securité sociale*" frequently when you arrive. I was confused by the meaning of this until I discovered that French social security is not the same as American social security. In France, it is the term given to reimbursement by the government for medical expenses. (However, a model must have completed eight work assignments in a month to be reimbursed. This is a law.) Each agency delegates a staff member to handle working papers for new models. This task is handled diligently. A breach of the rules will result in the prosecution of the agency and the deportation of the model.

American models do not need a visa to enter France. Don't forget to take your birth certificate to Paris! This is essential for obtaining official documents.

Your first task at the agency will be to go with the staff member to the foreign labor office and then to the police station. You will sign a lot of papers and submit eight passport-size photographs. At the end of the formalities, you will receive a social security number, a work permit, and a "*carte de séjour,*" which is a resident's permit. The work and resident's permits last for three months. A few weeks later you will take an obligatory medical examination, and if all goes well you will receive a six-month work permit. Then it's back to the police station for a six-month resident's permit. These documents may only be renewed twice and must never be allowed to expire. Think hard before you change agencies. When you do, the documents become invalid and you have to start all over again with your new agency! These facts strongly emphasize that one cannot drift from one European country to another hoping to obtain work.

Social security, mandatory tax, and some insurance deductions will be taken from your salary.

Models flood into Paris from all over the world for the Haute Couture (January and July) and Prêt-à-Porter (March, September, and October) months. August, however, is vacation time for the French and all model agencies close.

Paris is a city for all models, from the beginner to the highest paid. The large, well-established agencies teem with activity, and bookers sit with telephones at each ear, switching from one language to another with incredible ease. It is an amazing sight, and their knowledge of languages never ceases to amaze and impress me. The big agencies can be overwhelming for some newcomers who might be intimidated by the hustle and bustle. For these people there are good smaller agencies. This is something you should talk to your mother agent or school director about before you leave home.

Height requirements for women in Paris are 5'9" to 6' with occasional exceptions. For the Collections, a girl must be at least 5'9" and the maximum hip measurement is 34". Height for men is 6' to 6'2". All categories of modeling are available for both sexes.

In Paris a pleasant attitude and professionalism are as important as a good figure and face. Clients and photographers want to work quickly and efficiently. Time is money and tantrums are not tolerated.

Paris is an expensive city. New models should have sufficient money to support themselves for the first three months. For Americans that is about $1,500 to $2,000. At this early stage you will not have tear sheets. A few good pictures will be sufficient. Once you are working, you will need three portfolios. The reason for this is that clients are tired of mile-long lines and insist on preselecting models from books before the final interview. The messenger services' fees for delivering models' books all over Paris are high and as a result agents balk at the cost and urge their bookers to persuade the clients to see the girls first. It doesn't work; the clients refuse. This means that you will need your own portfolio, one for the agency, and one to be taken around Paris to the clients.

Having three portfolios is not only an expensive proposition but a difficult one. Foreign magazines are hard to find in Paris, so if you have worked in other countries, these foreign tear sheets may be hard to collect. Photographic prints are expensive. There are, however, good copying-machine businesses in the city and your agency will tell you where to find them.

There are sixty-five model agencies in Paris. I strongly advise you to check telephone directories for current listings as locations, telephone numbers, and staff members change constantly.

Here is one very experienced agent's view on modeling in the city of lights: "Paris is still the first market in the world and everyone wants to come here. There are so many girls here, each one prettier than the next. When I bring girls to Paris, I tell them the truth from the beginning. This is a cruel profession. Modeling is hard work for everyone. And I am very, very selective. They can't go to a disco on the weekend and show up the next day with bags under their eyes for a photographic shoot."

I asked her for her comments on the controversial "60 Minutes" program on the modeling profession in Paris. She said: "Unfortunately it made us all look bad. It only gave one side of the story. But really, I am happy about the program, because now everyone will be more careful. I do not want to say anything about specific agencies, but I do warn parents and mother agents to know the agents they are sending the girls to in Paris. Problems happen so easily. A girl should go to New York first and work through an agency there.

"There is so much pressure on a new model. Her agency should be like a family, like a second home. Otherwise a model's life would be impossible and she would go home after a few weeks. I feel very responsible for the girls I work with. I advise them, groom them, and mold them, and am very happy when they succeed."

Crystal and Bananas

Renée Dujac Cassou is a beautiful and highly respected agent on the international scene. She was a booker with prominent Paris agencies before opening Crystal in 1985. She believes that young girls should not go to agencies run by men. "Women owners are more professional. And they are less competitive; they don't take girls away from each other." I asked Renée what factors determine a good agency. She said: "Good agencies have 'stars.' They are well organized and well financed. There are sixty-five agencies in Paris. Only fifteen of them are good."

The Crystal agency starts girls at sixteen years of age. The minimum height requirement is 5'9". Several Americans are among the forty models. "American girls make excellent models. They are born for the media," says Renée. She also owns Bananas, an immensely successful agency exclusively for men, which has seventy models.

Agency address: 217 rue du Faubourg St-Honoré, 75008 Paris. Tel. 42 25 82 82 and 42 89 42 09, respectively.

Ford France

Ford France opened in Paris in March 1991. At the famous Ford Models agency in New York, Executive Vice President Joe Hunter told me: "New models have to go to Europe for experience. We used to send them to other agents in Paris; now we send them to Ford France. By having our own agency there, we feel we can keep control and know what they are doing. They feel safe there. From a top model's viewpoint, it gives us complete control of their career. It makes us better managers."

Commenting on changes in the modeling profession in the last few years, Joe said: "The height for models is much taller—5'9" is short these days. In the last three or four years we have seen a change in the diversity of the looks. Now there is much more opportunity for lots of different-looking girls. The melting pot of all the different ethnic groups has given us a more diversified look in fashion and advertising."

Agency address: Ford France, 29 rue Danielle Casanova, 75001 Paris. Tel. 40 20 98 40.

Saga Model Management

This agency has the power of many years of experience behind it. Owners Nicolas Fiani, Eva Delorme, and Eva Arany have been successful agents for many years.

Nicolas was an engineer and owned a publishing company and an advertising business before he turned to the modeling field in 1984. He has definite views on what it takes to become a model. He told me: "There are three important factors in the making of a model. She must first have the gift God has given her—the looks. Secondly, she must have a professional agency that believes in her. Thirdly, she must have the willpower. This is a serious business. It is also a tough, tough business. I see some girls make it and other girls with equal potential fall completely apart because they do not have the willpower to cope with the demands. They must always be beautifully groomed and always be on time. And they cannot party very much."

Nicolas emphasized that a model must be able to support herself for the first two or three months. He also stressed that it is not easy to get tear sheets and that it takes time. "The business has changed very much in the last two or three years. The standard is higher and it is much tougher for everyone."

Eva Delorme is Swedish and has lived most of her life in France. She started the original Eva Models. Eva is charming and loved by everyone in the business. Eva Arany is recognized as one of the best runway specialists in the industry. She has booked models for top designers for over sixteen years. Eva is also an expert at building new careers, which makes Saga an excellent agency for young models starting in the business.

Height requirements at Saga are 5′9″ to 5′11″, with some exceptions.

Agency address: Saga Model Management, 11 rue du Colisée, 75008 Paris. Tel. 42 56 47 47. Fax 42 56 47 48.

The FAM Agency

Fabienne Martin is the multi-lingual, cultured, gracious owner of FAM. The word FAM is a pun on the French word *femme* which means woman. The first two letters, "FA" (pronounced separately), are Fabienne's nickname. The "M" from her last name was added to create the name of her agency when it was founded thirteen years ago. Fabienne has created a special family ambience at FAM.

An agency representative said: "It is not the fast-lane type of life here. Our models are smart, respected, and exceptionally sane. We have some girls who don't want to do advertisements for cigarettes, furs, liquor, or lingerie. Some girls don't want to work in South Africa. Not all of our models are like this but we respect the ones who are, even though their politics may not be ours. We don't book every job that comes into the agency. We only work with the top magazines, photographers, and advertising campaigns.

"We never take on a girl from a photograph alone. It is too risky. This business is too competitive. We can't afford to take a girl who is not an experienced traveler, a girl who might be frightened in a foreign city. We have to be sure she is emotionally stable. This job has very little to do with beauty, it has to do with being strong psychologically. It is not about being on the cover of magazines, it is about going home at night and having a well-adjusted personal life. A model must be able to mix with people and present herself well. I tell my girls to keep their wits about them and not get into situations they can't control. Drugs are forbidden. We keep track of our models and know at any time where they are and their emotional state. We have a total of sixty models of whom three are men. The thirty models we have in Paris at one time have the luxury of being handled by five bookers."

Height requirements at FAM are 5′8½″ to 5′11″.

Agency address: FAM, 13 rue Washington, 75008 Paris. Tel. 45 62 58 35.

Zoom Model Agency

German-born Gaby Wagner is 5′7″. She has been in the modeling business for over sixteen years and modeled in Milan and New York. My first question was to ask her how she had managed such a successful career in those cities at her height. She explained: "When I started in 1972, the average height for a model was 5′7½″ to 5′8″. Then the girls grew and grew—and I got shorter!" This agency began a rapid expansion when Gaby took on partners Sylvester Beaumont and Natasha Goldman (of the now closed We agency) in 1984.

When Gaby first arrived in New York, she spoke German, French, Italian, and a little English. She now speaks English fluently.

She opened Zoom in 1987, a daring move for a young woman in a competitive market. "I knew the business from a model's point of view. I knew the clients and I knew the photographers. It made sense to open an agency. My background was a big help."

When I asked Gaby to tell me about her agency, she handed me her agency book and answered: "Look at this and it will show you how successful my agency is." It was filled with international magazine covers and tear sheets of her models. "Every model must ask to see an agency's book and judge the agency's success by it. They can compare it with other agencies' books and then make a choice. Sometimes girls are confused because the model agent or scout is a good talker and promises to make her a 'star.' Some people will place a girl with an agency because they are impressed with the charm of an agency representative!"

I asked Gaby for advice and warnings for parents and for models planning to go to Paris for the first time. "Some parents push their daughters into this career at too early an age. They must find the right agent and be sure their daughter is safe. They should try to fly to Paris and see where she will be staying.

"Girls don't have to get into drugs and sex to get started in a modeling career. I don't give out free invitations to parties to my girls. This is a serious business."

When selecting models, Gaby looks for very classic, very editorial, very special girls who are 5′9″ tall, have a maximum hip measurement of 36″, and who have good skin and bone structure. "A girl must be stunning and easy to work with. If a girl is stunning but doesn't have a good personality—she can forget it! A great personality is very important."

Zoom has forty-five models, thirty working in the city and the remainder working on assignments around the world. Age range is eighteen to twenty-one. Girls who are between fifteen and seventeen work during the summer vacation. The agency finds accommodations, but models are warned that rent is high in Paris and they must be prepared to pay $500 a month.

Agency address: Zoom Model Agency, 6 rue Monsigny, 75002 Paris. Tel. 42 60 01 36. Fax 49 26 08 73.

Partners

Husband and wife team Jerome and Joelle Bonnouvrier are two of the owners of Partners, which has a sister agency in New York. Discussing the Paris scene, Jerome told me: "In the last two years, instead of strange-looking girls, we have come back to more natural, feminine models with more voluptuous bodies. Claudia Schiffer is the perfect example, but we are not looking for a specific type of model."

I asked Jerome about the problems facing young men and

women starting careers in Paris. He said: "The main problems are generated by the new situation of being away from home and family in a totally new environment with a different language. The type and severity of the problems depend on the agency receiving the models. Models and their mother agents should carefully check the agency that will represent them in Paris. I think, however, that many models who are in trouble in Paris would be in trouble at home anyway. The best solution for young models is to feel the support of family and friends even from far away." I asked Jerome how long it would take for new models to a) work and b) make enough money to be self-supporting. He replied: "It could take from one day to never! On average it takes from five to ten weeks to work and three months to a year to make enough money to live on."

Partners represents forty-five men and sixty women.

Height requirements are 5′9″ for women and 6′3″ for men.

Agency address: Partners, 352 rue Saint Honoré, 75001 Paris. Tel. 42 60 33 00 (women), 42 60 58 90 (men). Fax 42 60 38 44.

Véronique Marot is another former agency owner in Paris who also has an excellent knowledge of the business. Born of French parents, Véronique grew up in Los Angeles and is well aware of the culture shock experienced by young people who have never been to Europe before. "They must be ready to come—ready to cut the strings with home. Also, Paris is very expensive and they must be aware of that. If girls are really serious about modeling, my advice to them is to find an agency that is run by a woman. Many agencies are run by men who like to have their courts of young girls around them."

Véronique stressed the high level of competition in Paris. "Certain things set a girl apart—good manners, a nice disposition, good features, beautiful hands, nice skin, good posture, and great energy. That is what it takes. But even then she must be patient. There are girls who will go on appointments for three months and get nothing. They become so discouraged. Then suddenly it clicks. Some girls don't make it for a couple of years. I remember once, when I was with a big agency, I sent a girl who I thought had definite potential to a photographer. But he called me and asked me why I had sent him such an 'ugly' girl. At that point I questioned my own judgment. Now, two years later, that girl is on television and everyone wants to work with her. She is everywhere. In this business you just never know when it is going to happen. Sometimes a girl's career takes off right away. This is rare—and if it does happen like this it often fizzles.''

There are numerous well-established, reputable agents in Paris. Here are some more of them:

Marilyn Gauthier Agency, 62 boulevard Sebastopol, 75003 Paris. Tel. 42 77 04 04. Fax 42 77 60 91.

Compagny Management, 26 rue de la Tremoille, 75008 Paris. Tel. 53 67 77 00. Fax 53 67 77 01.

Flame Models Agency, 23 rue Royale, 75008 Paris. Tel. 47 42 60 88. Fax 47 42 59 20.

PH One Models (men), Absolut (women), 50 rue Etienne-Marcel, 75002 Paris. Tel. 40 28 42 91. Fax 40 28 40 66.

Metropolitan Models, 7 Bd des Capucines, 75002 Paris. Tel. 42 66 52 85. Fax 42 66 48 75.

City Models, 17 rue Jean Mermoz, 75008 Paris. Tel. 43 59 54 95. Fax 42 89 22 65.

General City Information

Airports

There are two major airports.

Charles-de-Gaulle. About sixteen miles north of the city center. A bus leaves the airport every twenty minutes for the city terminal at Porte Maillot. The ride takes about forty minutes. There is also a train for the Gare du Nord station in the city every fifteen minutes.

Orly. In the southwest of the city and about ten miles from the center. A bus leaves for the city terminal at Invalides every fifteen minutes. There is also a train to the Quai d'Orsay, Saint-Michel, or Austerlitz stations every fifteen minutes.

Taxis are available and expensive. A bus service connects the airports. The trip takes about one hour and fifteen minutes. There is also a helicopter service between airports and the city.

Transportation

Taxis. These are always available and fares are registered on the meters. There is an additional charge for luggage. Other fare additions are posted.

Métro. This is the name of the underground train system. You can buy single tickets or a book of ten, which is called a *carnet.* This may also be used on buses. There is a bus, train, and métro pass, which is an orange card bearing the owner's name, signature, and photograph. The weekly pass is called *Carte Orange Hebdomadaire* and is valid Monday through Sunday. The monthly *Carte Orange Mensuel* is valid from the first to the end of the month. These cards provide very economical means of travel.

Now a word of advice. Paris is a hectic city and the Métro can be overwhelming for the newcomer who does not speak French. Take the time to plan your journey to and from your destination. It will help you to know that the destination given for each of the many underground routes or lines depends upon the most distant destination to which that train travels. So if you see on a map where you wish to go, by following that train route destination you will then know what sign to look for on the Métro. Write the information in a book (you will probably use the same directions over and over again) and have it at your fingertips. This quick reference will save you a lot of worry. Maps are confusing when you are lost, in a hurry, or in a seething mass of people. When you look confused you become a perfect target for underground robbers, of which there are many. So before you start out, sit down with your agent or booker, or another model, and plan the itineraries to and from your go-sees. Believe me, you will be glad you did.

Buses. Tickets can be bought on the bus. You may also use one from a book of Métro tickets *(carnet)* or one of the various passes obtainable in the Métro.

Cars. Vehicles drive on the right side of the street. If you do not have to drive in Paris, or anywhere else in Europe for that matter, don't. You will have enough problems and pressure without having to worry about hectic traffic conditions.

Currency

The unit of currency is the French franc (F or FF). One franc is equal to 100 centimes (ct.).

Banks

Banks are the best places to change money. They are open on weekdays from 9:00 A.M.–4:30 P.M. Some banks are open later and on weekends.

Telephone

On October 25, 1985, an additional figure was added to the beginning of all telephone numbers in France. In Paris the number is 4, giving local numbers a total of eight digits. To call international information dial 19 33 33. International calls or long-distance calls can be made from any post office. To call direct to the U.S.A. dial 19 + 1 + area code + number. To make a collect call to the U.S.A. dial 19 (wait for the tone) 33 11 and then wait for the operator to take the information. Parents calling Paris from the U.S. dial 011 + 33 + 1 + number.

Postal Service

Post offices are open Monday–Friday 8:00 A.M.–7:00 P.M. and Saturday 8A.M.–12 noon. The Bureau de Poste, at 52 rue du Louvre, is open twenty-four hours every day. Tel. 42 33 71 60. Postage stamps can be bought at a post office or *tabac* (tobacco shop), which also sells candy, film, and souvenirs.

American Express

There are many branches but the most central is at 11 rue Scribe, near the famous Paris Opera House. For lost or stolen cards dial 47 08 31 21.

Embassies/Consulates

Canada: 35 av. Montaigne, 75008 Paris. Tel. 47 23 01 01.
U.S.A.: 2 rue St-Florentin, 75008 Paris. Tel. 42 96 12 02.

Toilets

Look for signs bearing the words DAMES (women) and MESSIEURS or HOMMES (both words mean men).

Time Difference

This is Greenwich Mean Time (GMT) plus one hour; Eastern Standard Time (EST) plus six hours; Daylight Saving Time is in effect from the end of March to the end of September.

Tipping

The term *Service Compris* means that the tip is included. This is the case in most hotels and restaurants; otherwise, the usual tip is 15 percent of the bill. Taxi tip is 15 percent. Gas station attendants and cinema and theater attendants should always be tipped.

Water

It is safe to drink unless otherwise posted. Most people drink bottled mineral water, which is inexpensive.

Electric Current

220 volts AC in most places, although in the older buildings you will still find 110 volts. Make sure you have the necessary adapters.

Recommended Street Map

Plan de Paris.

Police Emergency

Dial 17.

13

Milan

Models flock to Milan from all over the world. You really have the feeling that this is a model's city as you watch them rushing from one appointment to the next, or sipping cappuccino in the Piazza Duomo (site of the oldest and most beautiful Gothic cathedral in the world), exchanging ideas and news from home.

Milan has more international magazines than any other city. This means there is a lot of work. The competition, however, is enormous. The superstars are here and thousands of other models of various levels of experience. In spite of this, Milan is an excellent market. A new model does not need tear sheets to get started; five or six good test pictures will do. In three months one can have a reasonable book, and after six months, an excellent book, superb experience, beautiful tear sheets, and prestige. A model who has "trained" in Milan can work anywhere. Not every agency has the time or inclination to develop new talent. A model who is accepted by one that does will be afforded the best possible start in the business.

There are three essentials for survival and success in Milan. First, you must have definite potential. This means excellent hair and figure, the right "look" for the market, a nice per-

135

sonality, and a killer determination to succeed. The second essential is a reputable mother agent who knows the business inside and out on an international level, and who has a strong liaison with, and knows everything about, the Milan agency to which she is sending models. The third essential is that you are emotionally stable. If you are very insecure or have a dependency on drugs or alcohol do not go to Milan. In fact with these specific problems you shouldn't be in the profession at all, certainly not in Milan. The city is full of pretty, penniless young girls who call themselves models but who have had little or no experience. Most of them are trying to escape from broken homes and colorless backgrounds. The price of living *la dolce vita* is high. They fall prey to playboys who pick them up in chauffeur-driven limousines and shower them with furs and jewels—and drugs. This sad situation gives the profession, and Milan, a bad reputation.

It is essential that you have health insurance and at least $1,500 to $2,000 in travelers checks.

Be aware that accommodation is a problem. Living conditions are sometimes shocking. Good apartments are scarce and expensive. Some agencies do have their own apartments or find pensiones or hotels to suit a new model's budget.

Milan can be glamorous and exciting. It is a fabulous city. The Milanese are warm and hardworking. Models are an accepted and welcome part of the Italian scene. If you are aware of the problems, and if you are prepared to take your work seriously and learn from the experts of the modeling profession, you will have a fantastic time and gain confidence, and the experience will be unbelievable.

Fashion Model Management

One of the busiest and most prestigious agencies in the world, Fashion Model has been in existence for twenty-three years and is one of the oldest in Europe. An energetic staff of thirty works in elegant surroundings. The business operation is completely computerized. Fashion has editorial, runway, and television divisions and a strong men's department. Height requirements for women are 5'8" and over. (If a model is really outstanding and beautiful she will be accepted at 5'7".) Men should be 6' and over. Weight and height must be in proportion.

Lorenzo Pedrini, one of three partners who own Fashion Model, explained that when Fashion takes a girl, she will normally work within ten days. If she has not worked by the end of two to three weeks, she is sent home. "This rarely happens. Our girls generally work five days a week. If a girl has potential and a nice disposition she will work, make money, and get a good book together. But if she doesn't have these basic requirements, I would advise her to change her career." I asked Lorenzo about the large number of would-be models in Milan who are broke and out of work. He told me: "The problems are not just in Milan. They are in every fashion city. The trouble is that these days everyone wants to start a model agency—in Milan, Paris, New York. Some of these people don't care about legalities. They don't arrange for work permits or pay the models properly. So, of course, there will be problems. It is the responsibility of the mother agent to check out the agents she is dealing with in foreign countries. She should know where she is sending the models. If a girl signs with a New York agent, she should be able to trust that agent completely. This is very important."

On the subject of the Milan nightclub and party scene Lorenzo commented: "This agency is concerned with business. I try to stay out of the models' private lives. But if they ask for advice, I give it to them. But generally they will end up doing just the opposite of what I say."

Agency address: Fashion Model Management, via Monte Rosa 80, 20149 Milan. Tel. 48 08 61.

Why Not Agency

I talked at length with Giampiero Paoletti, manager and international director of this agency. He described his agency as "trendy" and expects it to become the most popular agency in Milan. He said: "An agency cannot have a specific look or style if it is going to provide as many moods as possible for the customer. An agency is a service. I also believe that if an agency wants to have strong management, it cannot have too many models." Of the ninety Why Not models working worldwide, only fifteen to twenty are in Milan at one time. Of these, one or two are 5'7" or shorter. Referring to these girls, Giampiero said: "These are my little stars. I have been working on their careers for a long time and now things are starting to happen for them. I am happy that I believed in them; they fit the image of the agency perfectly." He added: "I love to find beautiful girls who are recognized as models immediately. But my challenge is to find interesting girls who are perhaps not so pretty but who have a great personality." Discussing the future of the industry, Giampiero said: "I believe there will be more super models, more beautiful girls, more cover girls. I don't see one model getting seven covers of Vogue, I see twelve different girls getting a cover every month."

Why Not has runway, fashion, print, television, and commercial divisions. There is no men's division.

Agency address: Why Not Agency, 2, Via Gioberti, 20123 Milan. Tel. 48 18 341. Fax: 48 12 966.

International Beatrice Models

One of my nicest experiences in Milan was an interview with Beatrice Traissac. Beatrice is a very caring person, much admired in the profession. Born in France, she has been in the modeling business over twenty years in Milan. She opened her own extremely successful agency fifteen years ago. Beatrice is always looking for new talent. She makes ten scouting trips a year around the world. She can spot potential "in a couple of seconds."

There are male and female departments and show, catalog, television, and print divisions. Beatrice considers Milan to be the fashion capital of the world for a model.

"We have so many fine magazines here and the quality of tear sheets is good. A model does not require tear sheets to start out and she can have an excellent book at the end of six months that will enable her to work anywhere."

Beatrice considers lack of money and insurance the biggest problems for models in Milan. "So many times girls arrive without a penny. They ask us for help. We have to pay for rent, food, and give them money just to get around Milan. They look on this agency as their second family—we can't see them in the streets. We should not be put in this situation. To come to Milan without money is a very, very serious mistake. A girl should have between $1,500 and $2,000, as well as health insurance, for her own peace of mind as well as her parents'. A man needs more money, because it will take him about two months to start working. Milan is primarily a woman's market."

This agency does not require a model to have tear sheets but does require at least five good test shots. If she arrives in Milan with a good book she will start work immediately. Otherwise it will take a little longer. Anyone under fifteen years of age will not be accepted. "We turn away a lot of fourteen- and fifteen-year-olds even if they are beautiful and even if they are Italian, living close to home. They are too immature for this profession."

Height requirement at this agency is 5'9" to 6'0" for women and a minimum of 5'11" for men. Sixty percent of the models listed with the agency are American. Beatrice told me: "Americans are very professional. But sometimes they arrive with a very superior attitude and do not appreciate the service they get in Europe. We sometimes take models who have not been accepted by an American agency. They are not at all grateful for what we do and behave very badly. They have to do something about this attitude.''

Beatrice and her staff are concerned about the welfare of their models in Milan. Each new model is briefed on agency rules and regulations, commission structure, the correct city map to buy, and how to use the metro. Suitable apartments or pensiones are arranged. ''Milan is a wonderful experience for new models. It is a school, a training ground. They won't make great money here because the rates for work are not high. They will make enough money to get tear sheets and a good book—and that is why they are here.

''I warn parents to do a lot of investigating before they send their daughters to Europe. They must watch closely. I am a mother and that is what I would do.''

Agency address: International Beatrice Models, via Vicenzo Monti 47, 20123 Milan. Tel. 46 92 599.

Jump Model Management

Dr. Gianluca Causa, managing director, and Marco Cabiani, director, opened Jump—a top editorial agency—on January 3, 1994. I met them while they were scouting at the International Model and Talent Association convention in New York, and asked them about the procedure for young models at their agency. Marco, who has a wealth of experience and great knowledge of the business, said: ''Beginners must be prepared to stay at least three months to familiarize themselves with the market, the business, and Milan. It takes two weeks to test and get a composite, and it takes two months to promote the girls. We advance airfare if we are really sure of a girl's success, and we provide apartments. This means that a model must cover her debts to the agency before she actually makes money.''

Jump represents about two hundred men whose looks range from ''the very classic to the trendy, very young, skinny guy.'' There are one hundred thirty women. This agency has made a major impact in Milan.

Agency address: Jump Model Management, via Settembrini 17, 20124 Milan. Tel: 67 07 0523. Fax 66 90 344.

Eye For I

Giuseppe and Patricia Piazzi, a husband and wife team, are the sole owners of Eye For I, which they started in September, 1991. Both have had many years of experience.

In answer to a question about what changes he had seen in the business over the past few years, Guiseppe said: ''The pace is much faster now and so is the turnover of models. There is greater worldwide competition, and this is good because it results in models' being more professional and more qualified. This is better for clients, the magazines, and the agencies.''

Giuseppe has this advice for young men and women who are starting out in a modeling career: ''Be strong. Don't give up. Be professional. Professionalism is very important. Learn about the business. Learn how to walk on a runway. Take photographic workshops. I urge mother agents and school directors to encourage new talent to do this.''

Eye For I represents men and women. Height for women is 5'7½" to 5'11". Giuseppe explained: ''There is what I would call a summer market for shorter women.''

Agency address: Eye For I, via Aurelio Saffi 29, 20123 Milan. Tel. 48 01 2877. Fax 48 01 2841.

Riccardo Gay Model Management

I asked Bruno Pauletta, the agency's international scout, what makes him decide to accept a girl and bring her to Milan. ''It is eight years of being a booker before becoming a scout. I know what the clients and the photographers want. I know this market from A to Z." Discussing the modeling scene today, he said: "There is not one kind of girl, not one look. The market requires brunettes, blondes, the very tall, and sometimes even the very short." I asked Bruno about problems facing young girls in Milan. "Milan is a tough market to start at the bottom, especially for a girl from America who doesn't speak the language. We take very good care of our models in Milan, especially the young ones. A girl must be ready mentally to come to Milan. If she is not, people will not work with her, even if she is the most beautiful girl in the world. They won't take the risk. My advice to girls who are not ready for Milan would be to first find another market in America—far away from family and friends, but still in America." Riccardo Gay has an excellent men's agency called Model Plan. Models must be mature looking, between the ages of twenty-five to thirty.

Address for both agencies: via Revere 8, 20123 Milan. Tel. 48 01 0322. Fax 48 00 5508.

Among a number of other excellent agencies in Milan is Italy Model Management, which has catalog, editorial, runway, and commercial divisions for men and women. Italy Models is the main sponsor of World Top Model, a European model contest that grows bigger and becomes more successful every year. Agency address: Italy Model Management, via Seprio 2, 20149 Milan. Tel. 48 01 2828. Fax 48 19 4081.

General City Information

Airports

The two airports are Linate, which is about five miles from the city center, and Malpensa, which is twenty-nine miles from town. A bus service every twenty minutes links both airports with the Stazione Centrale—the central station.

Transportation

Taxis. You can hail taxis in the street, but it is better to go to a taxi stand. If you want to reserve one, call 67 67, 85 85, or 83 88. Taxis are yellow. The fare will differ from the amount on the meter if you have extra luggage or if you are traveling late at night.

The Underground Transportation System. Look for the orange sign with the letters MM on it. This means Metropolitana Milanese. There are three lines: the MM1, which is red; the MM2, which is green; and the MM3, which is yellow. The subway is very easy to use and very inexpensive. Tickets are sold at newsstands in the station and must be stamped at the machine in the turnstile before you board a train. These newsstands close at 8:00 P.M., or 1:00 P.M. on Sunday. At Cadorna, the junction of the red and green lines, the stands stay open until midnight. You must have exact change to use ticket machines. Trains start at 6:20 A.M. and run until midnight. Special buses that follow the same route as the train run until 1:00 A.M. Bus, tram, and subway tickets are interchangeable. Weekly passes are a very economical way to travel. They require a photograph, which can be taken in a booth at a station. This must then be taken to the ticket office at the Duomo station where, after filling out the required forms, you will be given a travel pass.

Trams and Buses. You may use subway tickets on trams and buses. There is no ticket conductor to sell tickets, so you may buy these at newsstands or at bars displaying a yellow sign bearing the words "VENDITA BIGLIETTI." Tickets may also be bought with exact change at ticket machines at some bus stops. These tickets are validated by punching them through a machine on the bus. There is a heavy fine if one is caught without a valid ticket.

Cars. As in any city, cars are more of a problem than a convenience. If you do drive, stay on the right side of the road, and be aware that there are rigid parking regulations in Milan.

Currency

The unit of currency is the lira (L). Beware of all the zeros when you get paid. They can make you feel very rich!

Banks

Hours are 8:30 A.M.–1:30 P.M. and 3:00 P.M.–4:00 P.M. They are closed on Saturday and Sunday.

Telephone

A local call can be made with correct coins or with a token. It lasts for six minutes. For an additional six minutes put in more coins or another token when you hear the signal. Tokens can be bought at the cashier's desk at a restaurant or a bar, or at a machine next to a telephone booth. You can call many countries direct. To direct dial the U.S. dial: 00 + 1 + area code + number. Parents or friends calling Milan from the U.S. dial: 011 + 39 + 2 + number. There is a 24-hour telephone service at the Posta Centrale in via Cordusio 4. To place a call outside Italy, through an international operator, dial 15 and wait until you hear an operator. Be patient—this takes time! To call overseas dial 170. Again be prepared to wait for an operator. Tell him or her the number you are calling, then the number you are calling from. The operator will call you back when the connection has been made.

Postal Service

The main post office, the Posta Centrale, is located in via Cordusio 4. It is open weekdays 8:00 A.M.–8:00 P.M.; Saturday, 8:00 A.M.–2:00 P.M.; it is closed on Sunday.

American Express

This office is in via Brera 3. Tel. 02 85 571.

Embassies/Consulates

Canada: 19 via Vittor Pisani, 20124 Milan. Tel. 66 97 451. *U.S.A.:* 10 via Principe Amedeo, 20121 Milan. Tel. 65 28 41.

Tipping

A service and a cover charge will be added to your bill. Take these extra charges into account if you are short of money. If you are feeling rich and have had excellent service in a good restaurant, an extra 10 percent gratuity will be appreciated. Keep your receipts—you can be fined for leaving a restaurant without one!

Water

The water is generally safe to drink. In pensiones it is wise to ask first. If you are a newcomer it is probably better to drink bottled water until your system is accustomed to the change.

Electric Current

220 volts, AC.

Recommended Street Map

There are several good maps of Milan. Be sure to buy one with bus, tram, and subway routes.

Toilet

Look for the w.c. sign. You can also ask for the *toilette* or say, *"Dove sta il gabinetto?"* which means "Where is the toilet?"

Time Difference

GMT + 1, EST + 6, DST April–September.

Police Emergency

Dial 113.

14

Madrid and Barcelona

Spain is the fastest-growing modeling market in Europe. There is work for new and experienced models. The look for men is tall (minimum 6'1"), masculine, and healthy. Women must be at least 5'8½" tall, slim, and have a fresh, natural look. Models with acting ability do very well thanks to the large television commercial industry. The A.M.E. (Asociacion de Modelos de España) is the modeling association of Spain. It protects models' rights and controls fees.

Denise Cerezal, who owned an agency in Madrid and was an international scout for many years, had this to say about the modeling profession in Spain: "Spain is becoming a very important country for all business, including modeling. We have gained worldwide attention as a result of events such as the 1992 Olympic Games in Barcelona. Modeling in this country has changed in the last couple of years. Models must be more natural looking, have a good personality and a strong sense of discipline, and be extremely professional."

Her advice to new American models is: "Be emotionally prepared to work in different environments, with different people who have different working methods. The market in Europe is not the same as in the United States, so be prepared to change your look. Learn about Spain—the lifestyle and customs—before you come."

Stars Agency

Madrid is the center of the fashion industry. One of the top agencies in the city is Stars, which has been in business for over twenty years. It is owned by Bernardo Jil. During an interview in which we discussed the industry in Spain, Bernardo told me: "The business has suffered as a result of the recession. There is still work, of course, but the standard now is very high, and the competition very strong. Only the good people get the bookings. Even beginners have to be good."

Agency address: Sagasta 4, 2nd Floor, 28004 Madrid. Tel. 521 1111. Fax 532 2995.

Natasha's International

The oldest agency in Spain, Natasha's Models has been in business for over twenty years. It has offices in both Madrid and Barcelona and represents men and women.

Agency addresses: Velazquez 26, 3rd Floor, 28001 Madrid. Tel. 380 3643. Avenida Diagonal 469, 08036 Barcelona. Tel. 405 3435. Fax 439 5456.

Atlantic Models

Barcelona is the catalog capital, and fashion here is more avant-garde. The television-commercial industry is big. Lydia Mas, the head booker at Atlantic Models, told me: "Barcelona is a very commercial market. It is not the place for tear sheets. That happens in Madrid. This is a good market for beginners. They can practise a lot and make a little money. There are plenty of castings here.'' This agency, which is owned by Martin Ferrer, represents all ages of men, women, and children.

Agency address: Atlantic Models, Luis Munta Das 2, 08035 Barcelona. Tel. 418 8099. Fax 211 0591.

There are other agencies in Madrid and Barcelona that represent all types of work and have strong liaisons with agencies around the world.

15

Scandinavia

Norway, Sweden, and Denmark produce beautiful models. These countries are regular scouting grounds for model agents.

Sighsten Herrgardh, a Stockholm journalist, pioneered the business in Scandinavia when he opened the Stockholm Gruppen Agency in Sweden years ago. In February 1989 John Casablancas swung Scandinavia into the international spotlight when he opened Elite Copenhagen in Denmark. His expertise at model management has already been felt. Chris Havranek was with Copenhagen Models when it was bought by Casablancas. He told me: "There was great excitement when John Casablancas opened his agency here. The market really opened up and everyone became even more professional. He has really made a difference."

As most Scandinavians are blond and blue-eyed, models with dark hair, brown eyes, and a slightly exotic look are in demand. American men do well. For them, their "look"— which can be either rugged and masculine or have a boyish cast—is more important than their age. Height for men is 6'0" to 6'2"; for women it is 5'8" and over.

Norway, Sweden, and Denmark are excellent markets for local models who commute between the countries. Americans are usually brought in for prebooked assignments.

Chic Model Agency, Sweden

I met Susanne Östling, who owns Chic, during her first trip to America where she was attending her first modeling convention and scouting for models. She was impressed with the modeling school system in this country. She said: "In Sweden there is no chance to learn modeling. At my agency I train the girls myself and then send them to Greece and Milan to build up their books. Sweden is a good place to start a career. It's a difficult market but a nice experience. However, a model will never become rich here. It is more commercial and there is work for shorter models." Discussing the differences in the approach to modeling in the two countries, Susanne told me: "In Sweden modeling is not looked at as a profession. It is something that is done between jobs. It is not the be-all and end-all. After you become a model, you invest your money or go on to be a doctor or a lawyer. Swedish people want to become models for the traveling and the money. In America these things are important, but to become a model—that is what is really important." Chic represents about thirty models, male and female.

Agency address: Chic Model Agency AB, Södra Hamngatan 19–21, S-411 14 Gothenburg, Sweden. Tel 46 31 10 69 38. Fax 46 31 13 05 04.

Norway is smaller than Sweden and most of the agencies are in Oslo. Denmark is a bigger market than Norway or Sweden, and models make more money here.

Among the top agencies: In Sweden: Vastvenska Modellgruppen, B.O.S., Mikas, and Sweden Models. In Norway: Team and Elite (both in Oslo). In Denmark: Scandinavian Models APS/Elite and Unique Models (both in Copenhagen).

16

Athens

A number of young models I met during my travels urged me "to check out Greece" as a launching pad for a career. In Athens I found a number of successful and growing agencies.

Fashion Cult Modeling Agency

I spoke to Vivi Christi, an agent and scout at Fashion Cult, about the industry in Athens. She said: "Models come to Athens for several reasons. First of all, we have a lot of quality magazines, which means models can get excellent tear sheets here. Athens is a small, good market for new faces. Even if models have only two or three pictures in their books, that is enough. They don't need a lot of money to live here. Athens is safe, has a lovely night life, and has very interesting people. For ten months of the year, the weather is beautiful. The city and the islands are magnificent."

Fashion Cult represents men (height requirement is 5′11″ to 6′0″ maximum) and women (5′8″ minimum). This agency also finds accommodation.

Agency address: Fashion Cult Modeling Agency, 5 Iperidou Street & Nikis, Athens 10558. Tel. 30 322 1301. Fax 30 322 8281.

Other agencies include Unique Agence Models and Prestige Management Group, Ltd.

17

Tokyo

Japan is an excellent market for male and female models. Most of the work is in Tokyo. Every model who has worked there raves about it. It sounds good when you hear that all models are admitted to night clubs free of charge, and that all drinks are free, but some models have abused this to their careers' demise. In Japan, more than anywhere else, if a model does not play by the rules and does not look and behave professionally, his or her career will end quickly.

Japanese corporations pay their employees bonuses in the summer and at the end of the year. To recoup this money, they spend large amounts on advertising. That is why there is a great deal of work at certain times. The first three months of the year are spent shooting summer fashions; April and May are busy with fashion shows (there may be ten a day). Summer is spent shooting winter fashions. Japan is seasonal and models should make sure that their specific look is in vogue before they go.

The work routine is the same as in other countries, but the model agency system is different. There are specific rules, regulations, and requirements. Government law requires that there be a standard, guaranteed, exclusive sixty-day contract between model agency and foreign model. This contract can be extended for a further sixty days while the model is in Japan. The government also requires that agencies guarantee the following: a minimum amount of earnings for that period regardless of whether the model works or not, a prepaid round-trip airfare ticket, and accommodation.

New visa laws require agencies to have the government's stamped approval on all immigration papers before they are allowed to send contracts to models. Before entering Japan models must obtain a valid performance-by-contract visa. To do this they must go to a Japanese embassy or consulate and show their model agency contract with letters of authenticity; an agency tax statement on company stationery; three passport photographs; two composites; and at least three professional pictures.

Japanese model agencies take 20 percent commission and withhold an obligatory 20 percent for taxes. They do not use a voucher system, so a model should keep a record of money earned. There are no set fees for work, and bookers negotiate with clients. Payment is made at the end of the contract, before the model leaves Japan. In the meantime, the agency will advance an adequate living allowance.

In the words of one Tokyo agent: "Japan is the land of being accessorized." An up-to-date supply of accessories is needed. (Take plenty of shoes—remember, the Japanese have small feet!) A model should be met at the airport by an agency representative. Once in the country, models are taken to appointments by a staff member in an agency car. This overcomes the communication problem.

Models can earn a lot of money in Japan. Tear sheets are not essential, but they give an added edge in the increasingly competitive market.

There is excellent opportunity to work a great deal in other Japanese cities. For some models the pace in Japan is too demanding. One young American model was relieved when the time came to return to the United States. She was exhausted after her stay in Tokyo and found that the financial rewards were not worth the endless strain and pressure.

Folio

The Folio agency, which is owned by Japanese businessman Hiroshi Aoyagi, is an excellent example of the efficiency with which the modeling profession operates in Japan. It offers a $4,000 minimum guarantee whether or not a model works, and it forwards a prepaid airline ticket. The agency has twenty-eight apartments available all year. Since agencies must make four-month deposits on rented apartments, Folio spends over half a million dollars on rent deposits alone. Accommodations are exceptionally good. If two girls share an apartment, the unit will have two bedrooms, a living room, kitchen, bathroom, towels, sheets, and Western-style furniture. Models can usually pay back the money that has been invested and advanced within a working week. One day's work will pay for a month's rent; two days will pay for the airfare; and another day will cover food, electricity, and incidentals. Folio spends approximately $6,000 on a model before making any money. The agency must print composites, do mailings, and send managers to preselect clients and promote models before they arrive.

The Folio agency contract stipulates that models will be punctual, perform in a professional manner, obey the laws of Japan, and not engage in any other employment. The contract is terminated if a model uses illegal drugs. The penalty for being caught with one joint of marijuana is three months in jail and deportation.

Chaco Katori, executive vice president of Folio, is one of the most traveled agents in the world, as she is constantly in search of new models. We talked about how the modeling profession has changed in Japan in the past two years. Chaco told me: "It has become as competitive as New York and Paris. So many girls want to become models now." Chaco has seen the height requirement increase. For years, girls had to be short to work in Japan. Today, especially in Tokyo, models must be between 5'7" and 5'9½". A six-foot-tall model whom Chaco brought from London worked constantly in fashion shows, print work, and television commercials. Another major change has been the demand for the brown-eyed, dark-haired model instead of the blue-eyed blonde who has been popular for years.

Chaco is proud of the fact that Japan is a very safe place for young models to work and welcomes parents who visit Tokyo. Sometimes there are problems, however. She told me: "Models are treated like princesses and sometimes it goes to their heads. The food and drinks are free in discos. We allow them to go there until 10 P.M. at the very latest. We check the discos at 11 P.M. to make sure the girls are not there. If they disobey, we give them three warnings. Then we send them home. I am very strict with the models. I have a big responsibility. New freedom and being away from home for the first time can really change a girl. It is very sad."

Chaco added this piece of advice: "Japanese clients love perfect skin. Models must take care of their skin. They can't work if they have wrinkles or skin imperfections. And freckles are out."

Chaco showed me the orientation package that is given to each model on arrival. Agency procedures and rules are laid out clearly, and detailed maps guide models to assignment locations. New models are taken around Tokyo by managers in agency cars until they are familiar with the transportation system. Under Folio's wing, a young girl can have a challenging, educational, and extremely lucrative stay in Japan.

Here is one example of an overnight success story. Erin Gastineau of Arizona was sixteen when she first went to Japan. She was discovered by a representative of the Folio agency at a modeling convention here in the United States. She was not a competitor but a member of the staff working at the competition. Folio gave her a sixty-day contract and a $4,000 minimum guarantee. Within seven weeks Erin had netted $26,000. Blonde, 5'6" tall, fine-boned, and weighing one hundred pounds, she was perfect for Japan. Erin is very bright. Though she had dropped out of the second semester of her junior year at high school, she kept up her studies through correspondence and by the time she returned to America she was ready for her senior year. During her stay she learned to speak Japanese, and when she came home she studied investments with her accountant father. Her mother, Christie Gastineau, said: "Japan was Erin's first time away from home. She experienced culture shock but it didn't last long. She traveled all over Japan and learned a great deal in a short time. Erin was lucky. She got it all right at the beginning—very much by accident!"

Erin returned to model in Japan seven times in the next two years.

Agency address: Folio, 3-16-15 Roppongi, ·Minato-Ku, Tokyo 106. Tel. 03 3586 6481. Fax 03 3505 2980.

Yoshié Inc.

Yoshura Furuya has owned this agency for thirteen years and has been in the business for over twenty. She told me: "In the past couple of years, the market has been influenced by the recession. The demand is smaller now and an agency must be very sure that a model will work." Age range for this agency is sixteen to twenty-four; height 5'7" (5'6" in some cases) to 5'9".

Agency address: Yoshié Inc., #302 K's Apartment 4-30-22, Taishido, Setagayu-ku, Tokyo 154. Tel. 03 5481 2224. Fax 03 5481 5832.

Model Chic

Agency president Tsutomu Oki explained the government's agency contract rule: "The government does not want us to bring in anyone who will not work. This protects the model from unemployment. The guarantee will pay back what they owe for airfare, apartments, and other expenses. However, if we offer someone ten thousand dollars we believe that they are going to book twenty or fifty thousand dollars and more. At Chic we only take models who will meet the qualifications of the Japanese market.''

Age range is fifteen to twenty. Height for women is 5′7″ to 5′9½″; for men: 5′11″ to 6′2″.

Agency address: Model Chic Co. Ltd., Rm 702 Anx. Harajuku New, Sky Heights 3-52-5 Sendagaya, Shibuya-ku, Tokyo 151. Tel. 03 3478 5867. Fax 03 3478 5895.

Male models also have great success in Japan. Phillip Brecker, an American, is one of them. He is represented by agencies in New York, San Francisco, Germany, and Milan. In Tokyo he is with Friday's Model Agency.

According to Phillip, ''Japan is an excellent experience and a good place to start. Modeling in Japan is treated as a high-powered business. You are expected to be very professional. There is a lot of work here and the night life is great. But drugs are a definite no. It is stricter here than anywhere.''

Phillip is typical of the men who model in Japan. They work, have a great time, and make money they invest well. Competition has soared in the last few years, and a good book with tear sheets from America and Italy is a great advantage. Height requirement is 5′11″–6′1½″. Suit size is 40 Regular. Clients use men who are slim and good-looking. They do not like the bodybuilder image.

Cyo Inaba, a Japanese actress and model, and an international model agency scout, summed up the modeling scene: ''The look in Japan changes all the time. The younger girls are the best. Guys must be slim; a big build is not right for Japan. There is so much work and it is becoming a very big market for foreign models. A model must have a pleasant personality. Clients in Japan want to work with people, not just faces. Models who are professional and pleasant will do well.''

Among other model agencies in Tokyo are:

Ad-Plan Tokyo Co., Ltd., 5F M Bldg., 7-9-7, Akasaka, Minato-ku, Tokyo. Tel. 03 5570 1168. Fax 03 5570 1154.
Team Inc., Shimato Bldg., 9-F, 8-5-34 Akasaka, Minato-ku, Tokyo 107. Tel. 03 3423 8311. Fax 03 3423 8310.

Tokyo is the editorial center for Japan. Osaka is the commercial and catalog center.

General City Information

I have been to Japan many times and can assure you that your stay there will be enjoyable and educational. Your agency will guide and help you. I have added this information section to show you that Tokyo, which is the center of the modeling profession in Japan, has basically the same services as any other major city. And although there is a great change in language and culture, if you read this section before you go, you will be enlightened, more confident, and when you arrive, home will not seem so far away.

Airport

There are two airports—New Tokyo International Airport (this used to be called Narita) and Haneda Airport, which handles domestic flights. There are many bus and train services into the city center and the journey takes about ninety minutes. I strongly advise you to confirm that you will be met by an agency representative.

Transportation

Taxis. Taxis show a red light in the bottom left corner of the windshield when they are available. Passenger doors open by remote control, so stand clear when the car pulls up. Meters record the exact fare and tipping is not expected. Taxis are hard to get and they are more expensive after midnight, when all public transport closes down.

Subways and Trains. Tokyo's mass transit system is fast and efficient. Names of stations are written in English and Japanese.

The Foreign Affairs department of the Teito Rapid Transit Authority (TRTA) publishes a beautifully illustrated brochure detailing how to use the subway. It is very easy to understand. Good agencies will supply these and go over them with you. You can ask for information in English at information desks at certain stations, or you can call 502 1461 for information. As in every big city, avoid rush-hour crowds. All public transport closes down at midnight.

Buses. The extensive bus service is complicated to use and to understand. Before you use the system learn it from someone who is familiar with it.

Cars. Traffic is fast and furious and drives on the left side of the street.

Currency

The monetary unit is the Japanese yen (Y). Learn the currency ahead of time and this will be one thing less to cope with when you arrive. Check the rate of exchange in advance.

Banks

Open weekdays 9:00 A.M.–3:00 P.M., Sat. 9:00 A.M.–12:00 noon. Closed Sundays and holidays.

Telephone

Four colors differentiate the use of public telephones. The yellow and green phones accept Y10 and Y100 coins, and the green phone will also accept a magnetic card bought at telephone offices. Blue and red phones accept only Y10 coins. Overseas calls cannot be made from public telephones. To call on a private phone dial 0057 for operator assistance. To book a call, dial 0051. To direct-dial a number in the U.S., the sequence is 001–1 + area code + number. To call an operator in the U.S., dial 0039–11.

Postal Service

Weekdays: 9:00 A.M.–5:00 P.M., Sat. 9:00 A.M.–12:30 P.M.

American Express

American Express International: Ginza 4-Star Bldg., 4–1 Ginza 4-chome, Chuo-ku. Tel. 564 4381.

Embassies/Consulates

Canada: 3–38 Akasaka, 7-chome, Minato-ku, Tokyo. Tel. 408 2101.
U.S.A.: 10–1 Akasaka, Minato-ku, Tokyo. Tel. 224 5000.

Toilet

Look for w.c. signs.

Time Difference

Japan is nine hours ahead of Greenwich Mean Time (GMT) and there is no Daylight Saving Time. The time difference can be really confusing. For instance, when you fly from Tokyo to Los Angeles you cross the International Date Line and arrive in Los Angeles hours before you left Tokyo—you actually gain a day.

Water

You may drink the water unless otherwise informed.

Electric Current

100 volts, AC.

Language

Some English is spoken. If you speak slowly, people will try to understand and respond. The Japan National Tourist Organization (JNTO) has a Goodwill Guide Program with over 16,000 volunteers who speak foreign languages. The guides wear purple-and-white badges for identification. They are most cordial and are glad to help with language problems and answer questions. Call 201 1010 for English-language information service in Tokyo.

Police Emergency

Dial 110 for police and 119 for fire or ambulance. Speak slowly. No money is required at a public phone—just push the red button before dialing. Another emergency number is 264 4347, the Tokyo English Lifeline.

18

Australia

Australia burst onto the international modeling scene in 1985. It ranks third for model earnings in the world. Japanese cities are now shooting big campaigns in Australia, and some of the leading fashion magazines are being published there. Fares to Australia from the United States and Europe are expensive; consequently, agents have to be certain that the models they accept have the qualifications that will enable them to earn at least sufficient money to pay back advanced expenses.

Sydney is the center of fashion and advertising and is, therefore, the city for print work. Melbourne is the place for catalog work. Models can make money in both cities. If they have tear sheets and obvious potential, agents will advance airfare. Otherwise models must pay expenses.

Height requirement for women is 5′8″ to 5′10″. But there is no specific look. The look for men however, is specific— blond, tanned, energetic, and muscular. Height requirements are 5′11″ to 6′0″.

Chadwick's Model Management

I spoke with owner Peter Chadwick in Sydney, where he has been in business for over twenty years. Peter took over the reins seventeen years ago. He explained why Australia has become such a popular market: "First of all we have world-class magazines and superb photographers. The weather is terrific. Models love it here, especially the guys who take their surfboards to the beach as soon as they have finished a shoot. And clients like to work here because of a combination of these things."

Agency address: Chadwick's Model Management, 32A Oxford Street—Suite 1, Darlinghurst 2010, Sydney, New South Wales. Tel. 2 332 2799.

Chadwick's agency address in Melbourne is: 37-39 Albert Road, Melbourne 3004, Victoria. Tel. 3 866 3231.

Vivien's Model Management

Vivien Smith is well known and highly respected in modeling circles around the world. She is responsible for bringing modeling in Australia up to international standards. Vivien has an agency in Sydney, Melbourne, and Brisbane. She opened the main office in Sydney in 1966. Judy Steeves, a scout for the agency, told me: Australia has a very high standard of modeling. We really only bring in top girls. We are interested in girls who want to build up their books if they are really stunning." Height requirement is 5'9" to 5'11" and the age range is eighteen to twenty-two.

Agency address: Vivien's Model Management, 43 Bay Street, Double Bay, Sydney, NSW 2028. Tel. 2 326 2700. Fax 2 327 8084.

I interviewed Jamie Downing, a young American makeup artist and hair stylist who, after working on the Ford agency's "Super Model of the World" competition, spent three months in Sydney with Vivien's Model Management. Jamie told me: "Australia is a booming market. Everyone wants to go there—clients, film people, and models. There is a lot of work and there is not the pressure of other big cities. Everyone is laid-back. They all work together, but they are not in a mad rush. People are friendly and really enjoy life. I loved working in Australia.''

There are several things, apart from the great amount of work, that account for the Australian market's popularity. Australia is an excellent place to get tear sheets and put together a portfolio. For most models, there is no language barrier. Australia is a safe place to work and live. The people are friendly, easygoing, and sincere, and the country and climate are beautiful. Note that the seasons are reversed—it is midsummer in December. I remember spending one Christmas Day sizzling in the sun on Sydney's Bondi Beach. I spent a great deal of time in Australia, and I also lived in the Earl's Court (dubbed "Kangaroo Valley" because of the number of Australian residents) and Kensington areas of London, where many of my friends and neighbors were "Aussies." They are fabulous people. If you get a chance to work "down under" (Australia is often called that because of its location—south of the equator), then good on you, sheila (or mite). It's a beaut! And that's fair dinkum! (That's Australian for "good for you, girl [or mate]." If you get the chance, take it. It is great and that's the truth!)

Cameron's Mgmt. Pty. Ltd., 163 Broughan Street, Woolmooloo, Sydney, NSW 2001. Tel. 2 358 6433.

Chic Models, 155 New S. Head Rd., Edgecliff, Sydney, NSW 2027. Tel. 2 328 6900.

Pamela's Model Mgmt., 4196 Military Road, Neutral Bay 2089, Sydney, NSW Tel. 908 3022.

General Information

Metric

Australia uses the metric system of weights and measures. Temperatures are measured in celsius (centigrade).

Currency

The dollar is the monetary unit. One dollar equals 100 cents. There are denominations of $100, $50, $20, $10, $5, and $2 notes. There are $1, 50¢, 20¢, 5¢, and 1¢ coins.

Banks

Hours are 9:30 A.M.–4:00 P.M. Monday through Friday.

Telephone

Australia has a sophisticated system. International access code is 011; country code is 61; city code for Sydney is 2, and for Melbourne it is 3.

Postal Service

Post office hours are 9:00 A.M.–5:00 P.M. Monday through Friday.

American Express

Sydney: American Express Tower, 388 George Street, Sydney. Tel. 239 0666.
Melbourne: American Express, 105 Elizabeth Street. Tel. 602 4666.

Electric Current

The electric current is 240/250 volts, AC. You will no doubt need a voltage converter and an adapter for the three-pin plug outlets.

THREE

19

Specialty Modeling

Large Sizes

In the mid-seventies, big changes took place in certain areas of the fashion industry. The junior, or teenage, market had started to decline and the predictions were that it would continue to do so, even more rapidly. Initial studies showed that teenagers who had been born during the baby boom era and who had romped through their teenage years on a compulsive multibillion-dollar spending spree were now in or nearing their thirties, where marriage, motherhood, and budgets would leave them less money to spend on clothes. (Statistics show that a woman starting a family spends much less money on clothes than a teenager.) As the baby boom had been followed by a period of zero population growth, there would be fewer teenagers to buy clothes and, therefore, that particular market would drop off.

Meanwhile, there was a new category of clothes buyer in the store—the career woman. Studies showed that a working woman who earned $10,000 a year spent more on clothes than the wife of an executive who earned $50,000. However, although there was a noticeable growth in the career market, there was little hope that this would make up the deficit in teenage spending. Additional in-depth studies were done in New York in an effort to find other markets that would recapture the American dollar. One bombshell dropped by the study was that the fashion industry, which had always assumed that fashion-conscious women loved to diet and were rich enough to go to "fat farms" to stay trim, had been wrong. The shocking revelation was that 30 percent of American women wore a size 16 or over. Of these women, five to seven million were large-size women with moderate to high incomes, fourteen million had moderate incomes, and six to seven million were budget customers. The fashion industry was ecstatic. Here was the answer to the drop in teenage buying—an untapped and very lucrative large-size market. It is interesting to note that at the time a top designer who was ready to retire was asked to put her name on a large-size boutique line of clothing. She declined, stating that large sizes were not her image. Today, that same designer says, "That snobbery was the biggest mistake I ever made. I could have ended my career in a blaze of glory as a pioneer and trendsetter instead of ending it as just another talented designer. I didn't do it because I was a snob. I didn't know what the large-size woman looked like. In fact, she is beautiful and there are so many of her."

Manufacturers responded to the fashion-industry study by producing cute and elegant clothes to fit larger sizes. There was still a problem, however. Buyers balked, saying their customers would not look right in them. There had to be a way to show that these designs would look good on large women. A large-size model was found, and then another. The solution was a success. Buyers bought the clothes, and a new category of model was suddenly in demand.

Mary Duffy is a dynamic, vivacious New Yorker whose modeling career began in Boston, where she ran an art gallery and modeled large-size clothes on the side. Mary was Boston's first large-size model and was very much in demand. After some persuasion, she agreed to move to New

York, where her friend had opened an agency for large-size women. Mary tells her story: "I was making a lot of money modeling in Boston, but I had no right to think I could come back to New York and succeed in the business. I knew nothing about the modeling industry. It was a case of ignorance is bliss. If I had known what I should have known, but didn't, I would have been hysterical. I learned just in time. I became a partner in the agency and when my friend decided to sell, I bought her out and became sole owner." Mary is now a consultant at the Ford agency.

Large-size models are size 12, 14, 16, and 18. There are a small number who are size 20 and 24. Height requirement is 5'7" to 5'11", with weight in proportion to height. There are large-size markets in the major cities. If you don't have an agency that represents large sizes in your area, and you fit this category, it is worthwhile asking the fashion coordinators of local department stores to consider you for future shows. In the past year I have seen larger models in fashion shows in Canada and the United States than ever before. They did a super job and were well received by the audience.

There are several agencies in New York and other fashion cities in this country that represent plus-size models. I have referred to them in the appropriate sections of this book.

Petites

The results of the New York fashion market study that produced the startling revelations about the large-size woman did the same for the petite woman. It showed that the average American woman is a little shorter than 5'4" (5'3.8", to be exact—only one in ten women is 5'10" or over). This meant that a market for petite sizes could be as great as 50 percent of American women.

Virginia DeBerry, a former vice president of an agency for

petites, told me: "It is totally out of the question that a girl who is 5′3″ or 5′4″ will become a superstar model in New York. As long as big catalog companies can write 'also available in petite' across the bottom of a picture, they will not use petite models. There has to be a reeducation of the petite woman. She must write to the department stores and ask to see petite mannequins modeling clothing. She must write to the catalog companies and ask them to use petite models. She must insist that she be represented as she is—a petite woman. This is what women with full figures did. It became almost a political cause. Now it is a booming industry. Calvin Klein is one of a number of designers who are putting out a petite line. This company uses petite models to fit the garments, to model in showrooms, and to sell the petite-size garments to store buyers, but they will not use them in print advertisement—yet! But this will come."

I spoke with Mary Catherine McCarthy, who was extremely knowledgeable about this specialty, having worked for an agency for petite models. She said: "American women will not be dictated to anymore. They demand that petite models model petite clothes.

"Photographers often prefer petite models because they have better proportions. Height is only an issue on a runway or in a live performance.

"Television provides a definite career path for a petite model. Lipstick does not need height. Nothing in the beauty industry has anything to do with height. But a petite model must have a beautiful face and a very good figure. Acting ability is a great asset because so much of the work is in television."

Susanne Johnson, a Chicago agent who handles some petite models, said: "It is very hard for a petite model. She has to be very special and be prepared to travel a lot."

Mary Theresa Zazzera worked in the specialty division of the Ford agency for twelve years and is now a consultant to the industry. She told me: "Petites can do print work and they can work in the fit and showroom markets. Book covers are another aspect—many of the girls who work with Fabio are quite diminutive. Also, many petites wear a size six shoe which is the sample size for shoe photography. A shorter girl can make it in this industry, if she is prepared to spread herself more thinly than other models. As far as a major career? The Kate Mosses are the exception, not the rule!''

I have discussed agencies that represent petites in various sections of this book.

I met Dan Stanton when he was in the throes of developing *Petite* magazine. He was instrumental in getting *BBW* (Big Beautiful Women) magazine published.

At his office in Beverly Hills, California, he told me: "There are forty million women in the United States eighteen years and older who are 5′4″ and smaller. They want to know where to buy clothes, who the designers are, and a lot of other information. *Petite* magazine will answer their questions and keep them informed of what is happening in the petite industry. It will be fashioned after *Vogue, Glamour,* and *Mademoiselle.* And petite models will wear petite clothes."

Dan got the idea for the magazine from his wife, who is a petite. "She never knew where to buy clothes. I started to do some research and decided there was a need for a magazine."

When a client requests a petite model for a job, only a petite model should show up. I am 5′9″, and I remember going on a television commercial casting for an alleged luxury yacht. There were several 5′9″ blondes at the casting. The interviews became shorter and the casting director more irritable as time wore on. By the time my turn came he was enraged! I learned later that he had specifically asked for petite models: apparently the "luxury" yacht was on the small side and would have looked like a toy with a five-foot-niner towering on deck!

Parts Modeling

There are lucrative specialties for men and women where height, weight, and age are not criteria. Models with perfect hands, feet, legs (sorry, fellas, not you!), teeth, eyes, and lips have very bankable assets, and the sum of the parts makes their agents financially thrilled.

Hand modeling, for example, is versatile and lucrative. An experienced hand model in New York can earn from $75 to $250 an hour for print work. Daily television rates range from $325 to $650. Make no mistake, hand modeling can be as grueling as any other type of modeling. Clients are very specific about the hands that will show their products. A small hand can make a product look bigger and vice versa. Hand models must constantly care for their hands and nails (washing floors and scraping paint is out—oh well, sacrifices have to be made!).

If you feel you could be a parts model, you may send photographs to the Parts agency in New York. Address for Parts is: Box 7529, FDR Station, New York, NY 10150. If you have potential an interview will be arranged.

20

Children

I have watched many casting directors and model agents judge child actors and models at competitions and conventions. I have attended many casting sessions. The child who is natural, polite, well-disciplined, and who can follow directions is at a great advantage. A child who pouts and refuses to do what he or she is told at home will probably behave the same way with a casting director or a model agent—but only once.

Many children are either too shy or too outgoing when confronted by an agent or a camera. The child who gets the job is somewhere in between.

Careers must be supervised very closely. Children should never be dropped off at a photographic shoot or casting. If they don't get a job, be lighthearted about it; rejection isn't easy at any age. If they are successful, try to take it in your stride without too much attention—this will take away the pressure of having to be successful next time.

As the mother of a child who did several national television commercials during grade and junior high school, I am aware that taking a child out of school for an audition is a difficult decision if it happens very often. Studies are important. So are school activities. It is very stressful for a child who is a cheerleader or a member of a baseball or swim team to miss a game or practice to answer the call of showbiz. They are torn between team spirit and school commitment and the glamour of being in a television commercial. And let's face it, the money earned on television beats cutting the neighborhood lawns for pocket money any day!

It is up to the parent to keep a good balance. A legitimate casting for a national commercial could result in a major contribution to college tuition and is certainly worth the time.

To start your child in the business you need a couple of Polaroid pictures: a smiling head shot (don't worry if a tooth is missing—it could be a $100,000 gap!) and a full-length shot in a favorite outfit. A little boy with tousled hair, shorts, sneakers, T-shirt, and a toothy grin will have the edge over a boy in a suit, tie, and sleek hairdo, unless this is what is called for. Send the pictures to a local agent. If the agent is interested, you may be asked to have a few professional shots taken. *Never* spend money on a portfolio for a baby or a young child. The pictures in your wallet will do just fine.

Here is another tip: if the children are taking part in a runway competition, don't try to teach them how to walk and turn like professional adult models. And don't dress them up in starchy outfits they have never worn before and will never wear again. Let them be natural, and dress them in something attractive and comfortable. Allow children to be children—on the runway, in front of the camera, or onstage.

I asked one New York agent to compare a child model's professional life with that of an adult. She said: "We have a different set of problems with children. With the exception of rejection, which is the same for both age groups, one of our biggest problems is having to deal with parents who want the business more than their child does. It is what they wanted to do when they were young. Children should never be made to feel that getting a certain commercial or print job is a matter of life or death. It should be fun for them, and when it ceases to be fun, they should be out of the business."

Fontaine Kidz

Jeff Morrone, an energetic, enthusiastic, and charming young man, started this division at the Fontaine Model Agency in Los Angeles. Jeff has specific information and advice for parents and children: "The quickest way to determine if a child doesn't have the desire to be in the business is if he cries when he knows he has an audition, or if she fusses and has to be taken out to eat and coaxed to go. This usually means that the desire is the parents' and I would tell these parents to back off.

"A third of the market now is children. The biggest demand is for boys ten to sixteen years of age. We look for good-looking boys and girls with lots of energy, ranging in age from four to eighteen. The best way for parents to get their kids started is to send me snapshots and include a stamped, self-addressed envelope. If I am interested, I will follow up with a phone call. The next step would be to come out to L.A. for a month or two to audition. If I bring someone in from out of state, I take them step by step into the industry. I help them find reasonable housing in a community where there are hundreds of parents doing the same thing.

"I would also advise parents who are looking for an agent to make sure that the agency does not have too many children—especially of the age of their child. Parents want to be sure that their child will get private attention and lots of exposure."

Agency address: Fontaine Kidz, 9255 Sunset Blvd., Los Angeles, CA 90069. Tel. (310) 285-0545. Fax (310) 285-9503.

I found the people who are responsible for building children's careers to be extremely caring. Two such people, Coretha Timko and Michael Harrah, are personal managers in Los Angeles who consult and direct workshops for young adults and children. Coretha had this to say: "One of the things we gripe about is girls trying to look older than they are when the business wants them to look as young as possible. Sometimes a parent will call us and say they have an extremely talented teenage daughter who looks very young. We ask them to bring her to get the message through that she must look as young as possible. When the child comes in she's wearing blush, mascara, lipstick, and a hairstyle that is unbelievable. It's hilarious!'' Coretha also emphasized how important it is that the child desire the career. She said: "When we talk with them one on one, without a parent around, we know if it is something they are excited about.''

Michael had this to say: "There are opportunities for children we never dreamed of ten years ago. The whole market is expanding and we are returning to family entertainment. We are looking for boys and girls who look like real boys and girls; who don't have a slickness to them that prevents them from being believable as the kid next door, or the bad boy in class, or the street kid that has had to grow up on his own. The child must want to do this with a vengeance, and the parent must be supportive. It is going to be a huge commitment not only for the child or parent but for any other family member involved. It changes your life completely.'' Coretha added: "We are interested in personality as well as looks. Sometimes a dynamite four-year-old becomes introverted at six. You would be surprised how often that happens.''

Address for workshop information: CMT Management/ JLO West, P.O. Box 3981, Torrance, CA 90510. Tel. (310) 316-0304, or P.O. Box 8892, Universal City, CA 91608. Tel. (818) 760-1895.

There are many other children's agencies around the country, especially in Chicago, Dallas, Los Angeles, Phoenix, Atlanta, Orlando, and Miami.

21
Advice from Models

The models with whom I spoke, from beginners to superstars, had different stories to tell about how they got started
in the business and how it had treated them. A consistent
thread of information came through in every interview. To
succeed as a model you must be professional, persistent, re-
silient, pleasant, and strong enough to stand up for what you
believe. I was most impressed with the girls I interviewed and
found they were very willing to share their experience and
knowledge with newcomers. Here are some of their stories.

Carol Alt

Cover model Carol Alt is a superstar with the famous Elite
agency in New York. She is an outstanding role model for
young girls. Carol is charming, warm, completely unassum-
ing, and very professional. It is obvious that she enjoys her
work. Carol's rise to fame is virtually an overnight success
story. Some years ago, on the first day at her agency, she
was told she had to lose 12 pounds. She weighed 145 pounds
(she is now 30 pounds slimmer) and was "just a shade under
5'10"." On her first go-see that same day, the lady who

interviewed her told her, in Carol's words: "Everything was wrong with me, from my head to my feet!" A photographer and a makeup artist who were at the studio, however, did not agree and insisted she stay while they worked with her. The happy and phenomenal ending to the story is that not only did she get the job, but the shoot also resulted in 92 tear sheets, her first trip to Europe, and the cover of Italian *Bazaar*!

Carol has learned much from her experience as a model and world traveler. I was present when she generously shared this knowledge with over seven hundred prospective models and parents at a modeling convention. Her mother, Mrs. Muriel Alt, who also modeled at one time, shared the stage with her daughter and passed on invaluable tips to mothers. Carol told her enthusiastic audience, "Don't ever compromise. If you have a gut feeling that something isn't right, don't do it! Don't do something that will come back to haunt you. Don't have a picture taken that you wouldn't want to show your mom and dad or, eventually, your own children." When a girl in the audience asked her if she had ever been discouraged to the point of giving up, Carol looked at her mother and replied: "Ask my mom how many nights I cried!" Another girl asked her how she felt about her success and her beauty. Carol answered: "I never really thought about being successful. I know that one day I felt I must be doing something right when someone asked me for my opinion about something on the set. . . . And I certainly never thought I was beautiful." Carol constantly stresses the need for professionalism. She considers it the most important characteristic for a model.

Carol is married to hockey star Ron Greschner. She attributes much of her success to family support. She told the girls at the convention: "Go to your mother and cry if you need to. Get it all out. You will feel a heck of a lot better. I was fortunate to have strong support from my family."

Mrs. Alt has this advice for mothers: "Have confidence in your judgment. Believe that the way you raised your children will pay off. Your standards will be theirs. Believe that!" I asked Mrs. Alt what her feelings were when Carol started her professional career. She told me: "I was too busy raising four children to pipe-dream. I was just afraid that Carol might nose-dive. I didn't want her to be hurt. Now it is so wonderful to see her channeling her energies into something she enjoys. She works hard, but she loves what she is doing."

Carol's sister, Christine, is a striking blonde with incredible blue eyes. The Alts are a wonderful family whose strong support has been a major factor in Carol's million-dollar success story.

Ronnie Carol

An exquisite New York beauty who now lives with her family in Los Angeles, Ronnie is a perfect example that success does not have to spoil the person. She is loved by the young people who attend her seminars on the modeling business. Her career began the day she popped into the Ford agency on her way home from high school in New York to see what her chances were of becoming a model. *She was accepted immediately.* Ronnie told me, "I can remember being so stunned. I ran home to tell my mom, and she couldn't believe it either."

Ronnie stayed with the Ford agency for twelve years and traveled all over the world on assignments. "I learned so much from Eileen Ford," she told me. "Being in Europe as a Ford model meant I was treated like royalty. I was invited to parties on fabulous yachts and in beautiful homes, but there was always a group of about fifty girls invited. There were no problems. The people who gave the parties were agency contacts and friends of Eileen. They never stepped out of line. They knew that if they did, Eileen would be on their case immediately."

During those years Ronnie lived in New York and went abroad on direct bookings only. Her looks, beauty, and natural ability to model made her an instant success. She did not have to spend time getting tear sheets in Europe as most models do today.

Ronnie has also had experience in the executive side of business. She was president of Elite Model Management in Los Angeles for two and a half years and knows the profession from all angles. In addition to this she is one of the few high-fashion models who has had a successful commercial and acting career.

Shailah Edmonds

It is an absolute joy to watch Shailah on a runway, whether on a video, teaching a workshop, or in a fashion show. It is an even greater pleasure to interview her. She is always smiling, and is the very best at what she does. Shailah is a top international model. Here is her advice: "Stay focused. Stay humble. Don't be intimidated by other models. Show compassion for everyone—we are all in this for the same reason. Above all, from the moment you step through the door as a model, be professional. This professionalism never stops. If you are really serious about being a fashion model, practice your walk and runway technique for two or three hours a day."

Shailah is one of a number of highly successful African-American models. She has produced an excellent video that teaches walking and runway techniques. It is called *How to Be a Successful Runway Model* and is available at Models Mart, 42 West 38th Street, Suite 802, New York, NY 10018. Tel. (212) 944 0638 or (800) 223-1254. Fax (212) 869-3287.

Gloria Dare

Another extremely successful model who is always willing to share the secrets of her success is Gloria Dare. She has a wealth of knowledge and experience from which to draw, having worked as a fashion model in Rome, Paris, Milan,

Zurich, and Hong Kong. She is also in constant demand for designer collections in New York and national advertisements. Her clients include: Revlon, Maybelline, Dupont, J. C. Penney, Oscar de la Renta, Revillon Furs, Charles of the Ritz, and Lily of France.

Gloria was introduced to modeling when she was fifteen years old. "My mother enrolled me in a modeling course to get me out of the trees—I was such a tomboy," she says. Originally she was with the Wilhelmina Model Agency in New York, and her first four years were spent traveling to and from Europe, where she did the Collections. She worked constantly and her portfolio was always up-to-date. During the next four years she did a lot of commercial work, which she enjoyed immensely. She explained, "I feel more comfortable doing commercial work. I don't have to worry about tear sheets and it is much more lucrative."

Though her hectic schedule no longer affords her much time to teach her popular runway seminars, she definitely has the knack of imparting knowledge to young people. I have seen her working with girls showing them how to walk and turn. She has endless patience and it pays off. She makes the girls come alive and move beautifully, making the clothes they are wearing take on new meaning. The thrust of her basic teaching is attitude and energy. She told me: "I can teach the basic turns, and walk and show the students hand and shoulder movements, but I can't program them on how to act on a runway. A model has to have imagination and be able to change her mood to suit the outfit. I show her all the options of movement. A runway model must always be aware that she is selling clothes. It is her job to make the audience go out and buy the outfits she is showing and make fashion editors want to feature them in their magazines. Their attitude and the energy they project are all-important. The same goes for guys. The secret is to make it fun. Don't try to model. Just model."

Gloria has this to say to young people who plan to pursue

a modeling career: "You will learn so much traveling around the world. It is an education in itself. But formal education is very important. If you are fifteen, finish school. You won't always have your looks, but what you have in your mind you will have forever. From a moral standpoint, if you find yourself in a situation that is not right for you, get out of it. Be strong and do what your conscience tells you is right, no matter what anybody else says or does."

Gloria, who grew up in Charlotte, North Carolina, adds, "Not every city is as clean and friendly as Charlotte, and Europe doesn't always have the comforts of home. Modeling is a tough life, but I am a country girl and I believe hard work never hurt anyone."

Gloria is a freelance model with a degree in psychology. She also works as a volunteer with terminally ill children. A master's degree in counseling, marriage, and a family of her own are among her plans for the future.

Sarah Webb

Although gorgeous Ford model Sarah Webb is very successful and has appeared in every major fashion magazine, her first year in Paris was slow and blotted with rejection. To girls who are planning to become models, and to models who may even at this moment be sitting in Paris, Milan, or London wondering if they are ever going to make it, Sarah has this to say: "Be patient and stay where you are. Don't waste money on airfare home and back again. It takes a long time to get established, but you will make it eventually. Don't make the mistake of comparing yourself with other girls. That can destroy you. I know it hurts when a friend gets a job you tried out for. But your turn will come. Remember, the client's decision had nothing to do with you as a person. Your look was just not right at that time."

Sarah grew up in Memphis, Tennessee, where she modeled during high school. A hometown photographer sent her pictures to the Ford agency in New York and Sarah received a call from Eileen Ford asking her to go to New York. Sarah told me: "Eileen said she wanted to see if I was really the girl in the photographs." Sarah went to New York with her parents, met Eileen Ford, and was accepted. Before modeling professionally, however, she went to a university and studied French history for eighteen months. But the urge to model became very strong and she decided to devote all of her energy to a modeling career. She was sent by Ford Models to the Karin Model Agency in Paris. The first six months were slow, with a lot of rejection, but by the end of the year Sarah had a book full of tear sheets and was ready to work in New York.

Her advice to young girls: "Always stand by your morals and boundaries. A girl who thinks she is going to make it in this business by sleeping around will be all washed up in six months. Sometimes a photographer will try to take advantage of her because he figures a new girl is naive and gullible. This is when she must make a stand and tell him she will leave unless she is treated with respect. Be very straightforward and businesslike. Once this is established there will be no more problems. They get the message very quickly. Always be true to yourself. This is a cruel profession and people will hurt you. But you will build character and become strong."

Tracy Matheson

Tracy was seventeen when she went to Europe to model. She had been accepted at a university and deferred her entrance for a year. Her goal was to become established as an international model, make money, and then return to the U.S., go to college—and continue to model. Teachers told her to forget the modeling and go straight to school. Model agents said college could wait; the time to model was now. Tracy struggled with the dilemma, made a decision, packed her bags, and left for Europe.

She was fortunate to have modeled for a number of years. Represented by the Dott Burns Model and Talent Agency in Tampa, Florida, Tracy had an impressive portfolio, tear sheets, and several commercials—three of them national—to her credit. She had earned her fare to Europe and money to support herself. This experience, plus the fact that she is 5′10¼″ tall, weighs 128 pounds, and has blond hair and blue eyes, meant that she had distinct advantages. However, if she was to succeed in this highly competitive market, she had to make the necessary leap from regional to international modeling and put together a European composite and strong portfolio.

It was difficult at first. Tracy found that understanding different customs, struggling with foreign languages, and leading the life of a fledging model on the international scene was a challenge. There were a few tearful transatlantic phone calls in the first month, but these always ended in adamant refusals to return to the security of home and family. Her resilience, determination, and immeasurable joie de vivre paid off. She did designer shows, posters, catalog work, television commercials, and acquired a new composite, tear sheets—and her first cover. Says Tracy, "I was lucky. So often I was in the right place at the right time. I remember one day flying into Germany from a little island off the coast of Denmark where I had been on a fashion assignment. I went straight from the airport to my agency. I had no makeup on and I was wearing a jogging suit. There was an important Swiss client in the next room whom I was supposed to see. I told my booker I had to wash my hair and change clothes before I met the client. To my horror the lady, who represented a very big company and an important account for my agency, walked through the door. She stood and looked at me and said, 'I want this girl just as she is, completely natural.' I was floored! On another occasion I had just arrived in Milan, and the Why Not Agency sent me on a go-see for a magazine cover.

My agent told me that although my portfolio was not yet strong enough for Milan, the interview and exposure would be good experience. I went—and I got the cover assignment. You just never know what is going to happen—or when.''

Tracy's career, however, didn't move into top gear until she met Sonja (Soni) and Ralf Ekvall, who own Model Team—one of the world's top agencies—in Hamburg, Germany. There was instant mutual admiration and respect. Soni knew that Tracy's classic look was the main ingredient for her success. She encouraged her to work only with this look and not change hair or makeup to conform to fashion fads or to please the whims of photographers—a mistake many young models make. Soni and Ralf have an almost Pygmalion touch in shaping and molding their models. Etiquette, exquisite manners, culture, and diplomacy are considered as important to a model's career as knowing how to walk, turn, and move in front of a camera. They encourage their models to become part of European life, to learn the languages, meet people, and understand the different cultures. The results are remarkable. By the end of the year Tracy had not only modeled in Milan, Paris, Zurich, Munich, Hamburg, and Scandinavia, but she could speak German, French, and Italian with reasonable fluency and had made friends all over Europe. Her stay had included a couple of memorable vacations—a skiing holiday in the Swiss Alps and a trip to the Greek Islands.

Tracy returned to the States and was represented by the Nina Blanchard Model Agency in Los Angeles while she attended UCLA. She is now a doctor. ''Modeling taught me discipline and perseverance which I found invaluable in medical school. The traveling I did always gives me something to talk about—besides medicine!''

Her advice to new models: ''Believe in yourself one hundred percent. Self-assurance is so important. Be friendly and adaptable—clients and photographers don't want prima donnas; they want models who are down-to-earth and easy to work with. And be patient. At first, you will think you are never going to make it. Then your career takes off. You are booked, rebooked, and prebooked. Suddenly there are new girls sitting around asking the questions you asked. Now it is your turn to console, encourage, and advise. You know you are on your way. It is a great feeling!''

As parents, my husband and I experienced a great thrill when we arrived in Europe and saw Tracy smiling at us from billboards and magazines!

Gabrielle Reece

Gabrielle ''Gabby'' Reece is 6′3″ and possesses a look that conveys both athleticism and beauty. She is often called the Veruschka of the nineties, and is considered a ''megastar'' by experts in the business. At nineteen, Gabby was an international cover model and a star athlete—the pride of Florida State University's volleyball team. In 1989, her sophomore year, *Elle* magazine named her ''one of the five most beautiful women in the world.''

Gabby was discovered by Coral Weigel, an international talent scout. Coral met Gabby when she was in high school and knew then that she had the potential to be a top model. Coral told me: ''I knew that no agent would look at a girl who was six three at that time. Even six feet was too tall for New York. And Gabby had to finish school. But I knew that Gabby was special. I knew she was star material.''

As high school ended, athletic scholarships came in and Gabby accepted one from FSU. During a summer vacation Coral decided it was time for Gabby to go to New York. One agent told me: ''When I saw Gabby and realized she was six three I told her she would either really make it in the business, or she would do nothing at all. She told me, 'Fine. That's what I expected. If it happens, I'll be very happy and if it doesn't, I'll continue to play volleyball.' She had a great attitude.'' The agency received major bookings for her for the fall but had to turn them down because Gabby had made a commitment to her volleyball coach and team. Gabby continued to juggle schoolwork and volleyball games to find time for modeling assignments. She spent her final spring break from college in Paris modeling for the famous designer Valentino.

In addition to being a top model, Gabby is a Nike spokesperson for women's cross training, a correspondent for MTV Sports, and a contributing editor for *Elle* magazine with her own monthly column on fitness and sports. Fame has not affected her outlook on life. Her advice for new models is: "Realize what is important to you in your life. Don't make modeling the number-one thing. Keep your career in perspective. Learn how to invest money, and get everything that is good out of modeling."

What a career! What a role model!

Beverly Peele

When she was thirteen, Beverly was spotted by a Los Angeles agent at an International Model and Talent Association convention. Within months, Beverly was modeling in New York and Milan and appeared on the cover of *Mademoiselle* magazine. At the time, I asked Beverly about her new career and how she was treated by her schoolmates. She said: "It was overwhelming to arrive in Milan. But it was neat. I was really excited to be out of America for the first time. My schoolmates ask me how I got started and what it is like to be a model. I tell them a little about it—I don't want to sound as if I'm bragging—and then I slowly change the subject."

Beverly is now one of the most famous models in the world. She is African American, 5'11", and represented by the prestigious Elite agency in New York. She has a baby daughter, Cairo. In 1994 they were photographed together for a fashion spread in *Allure* magazine. Her mother, Dr. Lucia Peele, assistant principal of Hawthorne High School in Los Angeles, where Beverly attended school, told me: "Beverly even took Cairo to Rome, Milan, and Paris for the shows. She just laughed and said, 'Have baby, will travel!' " Beverly was back on a fashion shoot three weeks after the birth of Cairo.

Beverly has had the support of loving parents. Her father John, a patent attorney, said: "We will do everything to help her."

Sara Olson

Nineteen-year-old Sara Olson is represented by IMG in New York, and other top agencies in Dallas, Chicago, and Miami. When Sara first arrived in New York she found it so overwhelming that she returned to her home in Cedar Rapids, Iowa, for six months before tackling it again. Her career was launched on an international level, though, when her mother agent, Mary Brown—director-owner of The Image Group in Cedar Rapids—took her to the International Model and Talent Association convention in New York. Sara told me: "Just because a girl is blessed with a beautiful body and face doesn't mean she can sit at home and eat. She has to watch her weight, exercise, and go on go-sees. A lot of girls won't go on go-sees because they are too tired. This is hard work. It's not about a limo picking you up at the door or wearing expensive clothes."

I asked her for specific advice for fledgling models. She said: "Be confident! Be outgoing! Be yourself! But if you are too quiet, agents will think you are standoffish. Realize that other people feel just like you. Always be loyal to your mother agent. Mine changed my life. I wouldn't be where I am now without her."

22

Male Models

The guys in the business are a superstratum of dedication, determination, intelligence, and masculinity. They are incredibly good looking. The dedication of female models is taken for granted. But men take the business just as seriously. They diet and work out daily. They read the *Wall Street Journal*, study the stock market, and talk investments. They model to make money—a lot of money—and see the world. This was one of the surprises I experienced while researching this book. I had no idea that modeling for men was such a respected, lucrative, and masculine profession. The good news is that a man's career lasts much longer that a woman's; the bad news is his earning power is much less. This is not likely to change.

Some men got into the profession by accident and treated it as a bit of a joke at first. But when money started pouring in and New York, Paris, and Milan became home they saw the potential for a financially rewarding career and world travel. They realized this is a serious business and that self-discipline and total dedication are essential if they are to succeed—even guys get bags under the eyes after too many late nights!

I listened to their stories with increasing amazement. Some

became instant successes, while others had to suffer initial months of rejection.

Scott Goodrich

Much can be learned from blond, ruggedly handsome Scott Goodrich. Scott was born in Atlanta, Georgia, in 1962. He grew up in military surroundings—his father is a colonel in the United States Air Force stationed at the Pentagon in Washington, D.C. After high school Scott went to the College of William and Mary on a full athletic scholarship and played football for four years. He graduated with a degree in psychology. Six months later he was modeling in Europe.

It all began in his senior year when he went to a modeling competition to provide moral support for his sister, who was a competitor. A scout from a New York model agency spotted him and advised him to lose weight and start modeling. Scott was 6′2″ and 235 pounds at the time—great statistics for a football player but not a model. With his football days almost over, he embarked on a physical fitness campaign. He ran five miles a day and cut his calories to 1,000 a day. He lost 60 pounds, thought more about what the scout had said, and headed for Paris. He had $400, no portfolio, and no pictures. Scott told me: "I starved for about six months and could barely make ends meet." But the starving and hard work paid off. Scott landed a major designer clothing campaign and never looked back. With his pictures in *GQ*, *Vogue*, *Harper's Bazaar*, and other major magazines, he is now in demand all over the world.

Scott told me about his weight loss and how his background and upbringing had helped him achieve a successful career. "First of all I told myself that if I couldn't control my own weight, I could not hope to control anything else in my life. I lost my excess pounds with a strict diet and a hell of a lot of exercise and discipline. When I was a kid my family traveled a lot in the military. I went to ten schools in twelve years! This made me develop great adjustment skills. Playing football for ten years made me very competitive. Discipline, adaptability, and competitive spirit are excellent qualities for a model. I model for money and that's it. I save 75 percent of what I make and plan to invest every cent. I have learned far more from my travel experiences than any university textbook could teach me. I don't sell books, vacuum cleaners, or refrigerators. I sell me—and that's one hell of a management job. I look forward to having a family of my own and my own business in the future.''

Keith Knutsson

An example of someone who has maintained excellent basic values, at nineteen years of age Keith was one of the youngest men to model in Europe and enjoyed phenomenal success. He put his modeling career on hold to go back to continue his college education. Keith is of Swedish descent (his grandparents went from Sweden to Tampa, Florida, where he grew up), but he looks more like a Greek god. He is tall (6'1½"), has blond hair, blue eyes, dazzling white teeth, a strong jawline, and a perfect body.

During his high school senior year in Clearwater on Florida's Gulf Coast, he had his first contact with the modeling profession. He was at the boat docks with his girlfriend one day cleaning his boat, when a representative from a large boat and sporting equipment company approached him and asked if he would take part in a publicity campaign. He told Keith that if he showed up the next day, he could ride around in one of the company's boats and earn $65 an hour while they took photographs. Keith was dubious but arrived on time the next day. "My girlfriend and I had a great time driving around in a boat all day. I made a lot of money. I thought it was a joke. I took the money, and as far as I was concerned that was the end of it."

His striking looks and great body were not to go unnoticed. While he was earning money during school holidays as a bellboy at a resort hotel in Florida, a model agent saw Keith and advised him to have pictures taken for a composite. His quick reply was: "You wouldn't say that if you saw my driver's license picture." The agent persisted, however, and eventually Keith had photographs taken and couldn't believe the results. "I just couldn't believe that was me in the photographs," he said. Once again he forgot about modeling, forgot about the pictures, and went to college to study medicine. His father insisted he concentrate on his studies and not work. Keith told me: "I had always had a job during high school to earn money to take my girlfriend out and have a good time. I didn't want to ask my dad for money, and he didn't want me to work." He remembered the lucrative day he had spent doing publicity shots in Florida, found the photographs he had had taken, and took them to a model agent in South Carolina. The immediate result was two television commercials and print work. About that time a scout arrived from a New York model agency and saw Keith. She told him he would be leaving for Milan the following week. He replied: "No way! I'm leaving for my chemistry class next week. Sorry!" As summer vacation approached, his local agent sent Keith's pictures to all the top New York agents. Ford, Wilhelmina, Zoli, Legends, and several other agents asked to see him. He told me: "I went to New York and saw them all. They seemed interested and they all wanted to send me to Europe. I was very naive about the business, but I realized I was very lucky to see these people, never mind have each one want to sign me. But everything seemed wishy-washy. Nothing was concrete. I was used to working with my father, a businessman, who liked everything to be cut and dried. I was so overwhelmed and confused I was ready to forget it. However, the Ford agency arranged an appointment with Karin from Karin's Model Agency in Paris. This is a Ford affiliate. This time everything was organized, and three weeks later I found myself in Paris!'' Keith was nineteen when he arrived—one of the youngest male models to work in Europe. He worked constantly in Paris, Milan, Germany, even Japan. ''That was amazing because I was tall for Japan. They cut an awful lot of sleeves out of an awful lot of shirts when I worked.''

After two years of traveling around the world and making a lot of money Keith decided he wanted to return to the U.S. and go back to school. ''I can remember the day I made that decision. I was shooting a commercial in Paris. We had been on the set all day, which was normal. Everything was wild and crazy and I thought, 'I have to get out of this for a while.' I wanted to be able to control my own destiny. I knew that if I went back to school I could do this.''

He started his senior year studying business at Emory University in Atlanta, Georgia. He chose Emory because he liked all aspects of the university and knew that he could model in the young, progressive Atlanta market. He especially wanted to ''blend into college life and be a normal student.'' He was obliged to have an answering service so that his Atlanta agent could contact him. This meant that he had to confide to his roommate that he was a model, emphasizing that he wanted this to remain a secret. This was not to be. His father arrived brandishing a copy of *Vogue* containing pictures of Keith; his roommate talked; and Keith's picture appeared that month in *GQ* magazine. The news was out. ''It was awful. No one would talk to me. The girls stood back and whispered, 'He's the guy in *GQ*.' Fortunately this didn't last too long and I was able to enjoy a normal life as a student.'' Keith became president of his pledge class and a member of the swim team. He quickly found that his experiences in Europe and Japan were a great asset in his business courses. ''I also really learned the value of money when I was abroad. My classes at Emory cost about $40 a class session and I knew I couldn't afford to miss one. Tuition is very expensive, and while my parents paid for this, I worked to pay for food, clothing, my car, furniture, and other expenses.''

Keith's excellent advice to young men and women thinking about or starting a modeling career is: ''Find out from agents in major markets such as New York, Chicago, or Los Angeles if you are right for the profession. If you are not, don't waste any more time. Decide on another profession. You never know how long your modeling career will last, so when you make money, invest it. Get advice about investments. Make sure you are financially secure outside of the profession. Exercise to stay in shape. Lead a good life. And don't ever compromise what you believe in. That's very important.''

A. J. Vincent

The lesson that can be learned from A. J. Vincent is that a model's enthusiasm and dedication should be placed ahead of financial consideration and the money will automatically take care of itself. A. J. is a refreshing young man who is a successful working model and actor. He is represented by McDonald Richards in New York. He knows his profession well and makes it quite clear to his audiences that modeling is a tough way to make a living and there is a lot of rejection. His personality and attitude are enthusiastic and positive. A. J. loves his chosen career, which is one of the reasons he excels at it. During an interview he explained: ''The male market has changed in the last few years. It has grown and is a very well respected place to work. But it is still the same story. If the budget for a job has to be cut, it is the male model who is dropped.''

A. J. has this to say to prospective male models: ''Go into the business with all the excitement, energy, and enthusiasm you can muster. Stay in it because you love it, not just for the glamor and financial reward. Your reward should come from doing good work." On the subject of rejection he says: "Rejection is a strange thing. You can try out for ten jobs and not get one of them. The client will tell you, you are not right—they don't mean you personally. They mean your look is not right to sell their particular product at that time. Then you will try out for a job and you will get it because you are absolutely perfect for that job. And they will tell you that you are absolutely perfect for what they want. It's a great feeling."

Fritz Sattes

Fritz is a great role model for young men trying to break into the business. I met him on his return from Milan where he had done some modeling. He had also worked in Miami. At the time he felt his portfolio was not quite strong enough, but he decided to test the New York market. "On Monday I was in New York making the rounds of agents. They advised me to go back to Europe for more tear sheets. By Wednesday I was in Athens!" In Greece the ball started to roll and before long his book was ready for Germany. He moved to Hamburg and his career took off. From Hamburg he told me: "I am staying in five-star hotels—that's how I know it is finally happening! I'm working and having a ball! I've lost weight, I'm running every day, and I have learned the language. I even had to learn to waltz for one assignment! Yes, the rejection is tough. But if you are determined, you can make it."

Fritz learned about his profession, followed advice, persevered, and is now enjoying a successful modeling career. This I feel is the key. You have to seek and then follow advice from the experts. If you have the basic qualifications, determination, a good personality, and a positive attitude, success is inevitable. Fritz is living proof.

David Martin

David has been modeling for seventeen years. He started modeling during his freshman year at the University of Iowa. "One of the sororities was doing a fashion show, and they asked me to model in it." David is a drama major whose career spans modeling and acting. Discussing the market for African-American models, he said: "The market is smaller for African-American models—and there are a lot of us out there. Any good agency will have representation for African-American, ethnic, or minority models. If they fit the criteria, there is a market out there. Hopefully, in the future, it will get larger." David's advice to aspiring models is: "Make sure you have an education. If modeling doesn't work out as you had hoped, you will have something else you can do. You can't be a dumb model. You have to be able to read those contracts and understand every detail."

David has modeled in the fashion capitals of Europe, but now prefers to work in this country. "I've loved the places I have seen. But I like being home in the United States."

Dodge Billingsley

Dodge still shakes his head in disbelief when he talks about his success story. He was helping on the staff at a modeling convention in Florida when he was spotted by Denise Cerezal from International Bookings in Madrid, Spain. At the time, he didn't have pictures, portfolio, or passport. The passport obtained, he stepped off the plane in Madrid a week later and went to work. There have been few idle moments ever since.

Dodge was born in Los Angeles, the oldest of eight children. His family now lives in Mesa, Arizona. His first brush with modeling came when he took part in a couple of fashion shows organized by the student government in Brigham Young University, where he was studying political science and international relations. He remembers enjoying the experience but thought nothing more about it. He spent two years on a mission for the Mormon Church, after which he returned to Phoenix. His blond hair and striking, rugged looks caught the attention of the L'Image/Casablancas Agency. Through L'Image, he ended up working at a convention in Miami Beach, where he met the people from International Bookings. The rest is a success story.

When Dodge arrived in Madrid he went straight to his agency, was given his first casting, got the job, and left that night for a three-day shoot in the Mediterranean. He didn't even have time to unpack. His first shoot produced a picture good enough for the front of his composite and tear sheets that were sent to the famous Riccardo Gay Agency in Milan. It happened again. This time Dodge was prebooked for a three-day shoot. He arrived in Milan and didn't meet his agent until the third day of the assignment.

I talked to Dodge during a brief visit to his family in Arizona. He told me: "Everything has happened so fast I just had to get home for a week to see my mom and have some of her home cooking!" I asked him if he had experienced culture shock in Europe. "I didn't have time. I went straight to work! But I was surprised when I arrived at Madrid airport and saw the guards with machine guns. I had seen them on television and in the papers but it came as a shock to see it firsthand. I have really enjoyed my time in Europe. I learned a lot about how Europeans see Americans and what they think of our foreign policy."

I asked Dodge what advice and warnings he would pass on to boys and girls going into the modeling profession. He said: "A New York agent told me that a lot of models go to Europe to play. When I got there I saw that was true. Believe me, that just doesn't work. It is a serious business. If I don't go to bed at night at 10:00 or 11:00 P.M., I can't be serious about working the next morning. You can't treat your time in Europe as if it were a vacation. When I am not working I study investments. I want to make the money I earn modeling work for me in the future. I definitely want to get a university degree sometime, but I plan to devote the next two or three years to modeling. I would like to be based in New York, but I know I have to get more experience to work there."

Dodge now has a master's degree and is represented by the top Nytro agency in New York. Dreams do come true!

Chris Havranek

Though he was born in Pittsburgh, Pennsylvania, his parents' home is in Lund, Sweden, where Chris studied international buying management at the University of Lund. His modeling career started the day he good-naturedly agreed to fill in for a model who had not shown up for a fashion show. A fashion writer told him after the show that he should go to a model agency. He took the advice, signed with Sweden Models, and began work. During the last week of a vacation in Los Angeles, he was seen by a representative of the prestigious L.A. Models agency who wanted to book him immediately. But Chris had to return to Sweden and school. He signed with a larger agency, Copenhagen Models (which is now Copenhagen Elite), in Denmark.

Chris's career underwent another surge when he entered and won a young-model contest sponsored by *Vecko Revyn* magazine to find the best models of 1989. As Scandinavia's "Man '89" he won a test with a top agency in Paris, a new wardrobe, travel opportunities, and much publicity.

Chris thoroughly enjoys modeling. I asked him how he copes with studies and the demands of modeling. He told me: "Agents in Scandinavia realize education is important. When they know I have to take an exam they work around it. So far, it has not been a problem. If I have to make a choice I would like to take advantage of the opportunities to travel and make the money that modeling offers, but I will always go back to the most vital part of my life—education."

23

Advice from Other Professionals

Parents often wonder if they have made the right decision when they allow their child to postpone college to embark on a modeling career. I asked the advice of many professionals and feel one fashion coordinator was right on target when she said: "If a girl is bright, she will always be bright, but she won't always have the opportunity to model. If she gets the chance, she should take it." Milan model agent Beatrice Traissac said: "Models are getting younger, especially in America. Even nineteen is too late to start a career." A New York photographer said: "At twenty-five, a doctor is just starting her career, but a model is a has-been."

One agent said: "Many parents are hesitant to let their child get into this business, but if a child has potential and wants to do it, parents should let them try. Keep the lines of communication open. A girl who has a problem in Europe shouldn't be afraid to call home because her parents might say 'I told you so.' It means supporting your child in a field where the chances of success are certainly not as great as in another industry, but the payoffs are tremendous."

Coral Weigel, an international scout for agencies here and abroad, has this advice for parents: "Mothers often ask me if I think their daughters can cope with an international modeling career. They worry and ask if their daughters will be chaperoned. I tell them that only they can be the judge of their daughters' capability to deal with situations and that model agents don't have the time to babysit. I also tell them that if a girl is mature and trustworthy, she will make it."

Kay Mitchell has worked for major agencies in New York and spent years scouting for models in the fashion capitals of the world. Kay told me: "It is always difficult when a girl who is young, inexperienced, and away from home for the first time is put into a new environment. She has to face a language barrier and all kinds of professional competition. Sometimes she does not react well to the city she has chosen to live in, or she might not be physically and emotionally in the right marketplace for her. Another problem is communication, especially in France and Italy. American girls are very serious about romance. They think that when someone is flirting with them, that person is in love with them. The French and Italian men just enjoy the flirtation. The Milanese playboys just like to be around pretty girls and know where the action is and who is in the modeling business. Girls shouldn't go alone to their apartments or get themselves into a situation."

On the subject of rejection Kay said: "Most of the girls who are successful are those who don't deal with this business from a personal viewpoint. They treat it like a business and realize that it is all a matter of the right girl, with the right look, being in the right city at the right time." She added: "I believe that this profession is an education in life. The experience can be transferred to any number of professions later on."

Television

If a model can expand a fashion and print career to include television commercials, he or she will become well known and make a lot of money quickly. Television commercials require specific training. Models who are normally comfortable in front of a still camera can freeze in front of video equipment. Here is an exercise to practice regularly. First, take a piece of paper and cut out a small circle. Cut out a second hole inside the circle about the size of a camera lens. Your finished product should look like this:

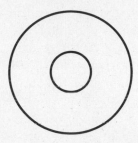

Tape the paper to a mirror. Stand about six feet away and talk directly to the hole in the paper, never taking your eyes from it. Make believe it is a camera lens and you are auditioning for a commercial. Write a thirty-second commercial or use one from radio or television and read it to your simulated lens. At first, memorize only the first and last lines so that you can deliver these to the "camera" without moving your eyes to the copy. Smile while you are speaking— this will give sparkle and enthusiasm to your delivery.

Randy Kirby is a multitalented actor, commercial casting director, and writer. He has produced over one hundred commercials for radio and television and has won a prestigious Clio award. I asked Randy for a few helpful hints for models who may be sent on television commercial castings. He told me: "The secret is to treat the camera as your best friend. Don't think of it as an object but as someone who likes and trusts you and will, therefore, believe what you have to say about the product you are selling. Once you have the feeling you are talking to a good friend, you will relax and your message will come across with sincerity."

Englishman Larry Conroy has a background in film, theater, and radio and has trained corporate and news media personalities. He has also "retrained" some of the world's top models, who, as a result of his expertise, combine lucrative television careers with modeling. His workshop, "The Model Speaks," is sought after by those who realize that today, being. able to act and speak on camera is a priority. Larry told me: "There is a great market right now for show hosts and field reporters in various cable programs. Models and other people with a good background in fashion are in demand. It doesn't matter how good your voice is, it's how you use it and what you do with it that counts. It's a fact of life—models need to be trained in this area.

For workshop information, you can write or call Larry at: 42 West 13th St., New York, NY 10011. Tel (212) 741-1444. Fax (212) 366-5688.

Leading fashion photographer Jacques Silberstein has a photo-video studio in New York. Jacques took time out from a hectic schedule to pass on this advice: "A lot of girls dream of being top models but what they don't realize is that there is hard work and frustration involved. I advise girls planning to work in Europe to check out the people with whom they will work. This is a new world for them and a lot of people want to take advantage of them. Models must be established with a reliable agent and have enough money to return home if life is not what they expected, or if they can't take the pressure."

I asked Jacques what a young girl should do if a photographer should behave unprofessionally. He said: "I have always told any girl who goes to Europe that there is no reason in the world she should do something she doesn't feel is right. If she does it once, it will never end. The girls who are the happiest in the business are those who are happy with themselves. A girl must stand by her own morals."

24

Plastic Surgery

Dr. Ian Matheson, a plastic surgeon practicing in Tampa, Florida, contributes the following:

"Plastic or cosmetic surgery can be a very useful adjunct to a model's career. Carefully think out the reasons for these surgical changes. Don't be talked into surgery by anyone. A beautiful nose will not ensure a modeling career. Other aspects are involved. Cosmetic surgery must be something you want to have done for you.

"One reluctant high school senior was brought into my office by her parents, pursuing the parents' idea of modifying her nose and turning her into a model. She did not have the desire, the discipline, or the dedication to be a model. The entire plan was destined to fail. I refused to operate on this girl.

"If you have all the other attributes for a modeling career, but your profile is marred by a nasal hump, or if you have bags under your eyes or a mole that spoils an otherwise clear complexion, corrective surgery could be worthwhile.

"The modeling industry is full of cosmetic surgery success stories. One beautiful blonde had a rounded tip to the end of her nose, and examination of her photographs showed a slight shadow cast by the sides of the nose. Surgical corrections resulted in a successful career and her reputation as 'the girl with the perfect features.'

"The camera can be unkind. Even a slight fullness in the lower eyelids (eyebags) is picked up. One model was told by a photographer, 'Your eyelid job has simplified my work—I can now shoot you from any angle.'

"At a modeling convention, a Paris agent told a fledgling model from Florida that her ears protruded. She came to my office and I made the correction. Several years later I saw the same girl, who said, 'The surgery was the best career move I have made. I never think about my ears now.'

"An otherwise beautiful girl with classical features had a birthmark on her right temple. When this was removed it left her with a small scar that could be covered with makeup. She was signed by an American agency and her career was on its way.

"Breast augmentation surgery is both common and successful. It used to be the number-one cosmetic surgical procedure performed in the United States. It has now been replaced by suction lipectomy as the most frequently performed procedure. Suction lipectomy is meant for people who are in basically good shape, but have one or two areas with an abundant accumulation of fat, often hereditary. The most common place for fat removal in women is the thigh and hip area, and in men is the 'love handle' and abdomen area. Models, however, must never consider this as a method of weight reduction but must learn to discipline their eating habits.

"Plastic surgery can be a useful tool, but do not have your nose, eyes, ears, breasts, or thighs altered unless it is necessary. Take time before you decide to undergo cosmetic surgery. Be sure that your surgeon is certified by the American Board of Plastic Surgery. Ask your doctor or county medical association to recommend a surgeon. Inquire around the community about his reputation. Ask to see the results of similar types of surgery and talk with other patients of that surgeon. If during the interview you find the surgeon cold, or uncaring, or unwilling to answer all your questions, find a surgeon with whom you feel comfortable. Cosmetic surgery is a serious step. If you do it, do it for yourself. Remember, a perfect profile or features will not guarantee a modeling career.''

25

Agency Instructions to New Models

Every well-established agency in the world gives models specific instructions on agency expectations and policy. Models One, in London, is one of the world's top agencies. With their kind permission, I have reprinted a copy of the information they give to their models. It is an excellent example of what it takes to be a professional model. Here it is:

Professionalism

1. Check-in time is daily between 4:00 P.M. and 5:30 P.M. Don't neglect to call in. If the agency can't get hold of you and you have a job the next day you could be sued if you didn't turn up! It's your responsibility to call us each day.
2. When checking in please keep calls brief, as taking up the phone prevents incoming business and that's how we make a living!
3. Keep a pen by the phone with your diary. Always be sure you know all the details of an assignment. ASK! Your datebook should also keep track of all payment details. Please also retain your model payment sheets and copies of vouchers to avoid any financial errors. Fill in

all the information on your voucher after the booking—vouchers are due no later than the Friday after the booking or they will not get invoiced in time. They must be signed by the client.

4. Always let the agency know, as far in advance as possible, days or times you are not available so they do not accept any bookings or make any appointments for you.

5. *Do not give out your phone number or address*, even if it is requested on contracts or application forms. Give the agency's number and/or address.

6. *Do not discuss business with the client* (rates or other bookings). Pick up the phone and call the agency or have the client call us if there is a question.

7. If (please, NO!) you are going to be late, call the agency, so we can cover for you. If you're late we will find out about it anyway because clients usually like to fill us in on these details! You should be arriving at least fifteen minutes before your booking time to all assignments.

8. Take everything you may ever need to *every* assignment. *Never borrow!*

9. A photograph is only as good as the model who's in it. A prepared model is a preferred model. Work your best with each photographer—you should never have to be told every movement. Practice in front of a full-length mirror to understand your body and its best angles.

10. Never apologize for lack of experience, appearance, etc. It only brings it to their attention!

11. Never argue with the client. They pay the bills. Even if you hate the clothes or find their directions foolish, be polite and charming.

12. In this business the most important product people are selling is time . . . so don't waste *anyone's*—including your own.

Remember

On go-sees, remember to take:

a) A–Z (A guidebook of London)
b) Portfolio
c) Extra pictures or card
d) Model's bag (who knows when you'll need it)

What a Model Needs:

Flesh-colored and black underwear (underpants, waistslip and bras) and a flesh-colored strapless bra.
Black court shoes [pumps], black evening shoes, plus sporty flat shoes.
Black or brown boots.
Good selection of makeup.
Carmen rollers [hot rollers].
Selection of tights [hosiery].
You should also have available and in good condition the following: strappy sandals, jewelry, scarves, sweaters, hats, berets, socks, belts, jeans, cords, etc.
Your booker will tell you what accessories will be needed for a job. If in doubt—*ask.*

When you go to a job you should always have the following with you:

Your makeup (even if there is a makeup artist there).
Tweezers, scissors, a razor, emery boards, absorbent cotton, cotton wool buds [Q-tips], nail varnish remover, tissues, cleanser, toner, moisturizer.
Brush, comb, hairgrips [bobby pins], and Carmen rollers.
Flesh-colored underwear.
A large scarf.

210

A folded umbrella.
A–Z of London.

Remember

1. Hands to be well manicured at all times.
2. Feet to be frequently pedicured.
3. Legs and underarms to be shaved or waxed regularly.
4. Clean, neat hair.

26

What to Pack

My husband questions my qualifications as an expert in the field of packing. He constantly reminds me of one particular train trip, through Europe, on which he had to rent an additional sleeping compartment for our luggage alone. Suffice it to say, "Do as I say, not as I do."

Extra baggage is costly and burdensome, especially in Europe, where models move from country to country on assignments. When packing, take into consideration the season and climate of the country where you will work. However, if you are going to be there in winter, remember, you will be modeling spring and summer fashions, and therefore you should pack appropriate accessories.

In addition to your basic wardrobe, here are additional items you should pack: a dual-voltage hair dryer and rollers; a voltage converter kit (this contains plugs for virtually all international outlets, and an adapter that handles appliances up to 1600 watts); a foreign-language cassette and tape recorder; a cordless battery-operated hair comb or curler; an alarm clock (preferably one that doesn't tick—if you don't object to the tick at night, your roommate might); camera and film; a sewing kit; scissors (pack these in your main luggage—they might not pass security inspection of hand luggage on international flights); safety pins; umbrella; slippers (European floors are often tiled and therefore cold); miniature clothesline and pins; pocket calculator; address book and an appointment book.

It is important to carry passport, visa, tickets, travelers checks, and address and telephone number of your foreign agency in a pocketbook or man's jacket. These items must never be in checked luggage. Make sure you have strong locks for your luggage.

It is a good idea to buy a model's bag before you go abroad, and you can use this to carry hand luggage. Listed below are items that should always be in your model's bag and taken on assignments.

- Makeup remover.
- Skin toner.
- Light foundation (1 shade darker than your skin tone).
- Dark foundation (3 shades darker than your skin tone).
- Loose powder with puff.
- Compact powder.
- Eyebrow pencils (+ sharpener).
- Lip brushes and eyeliner brushes.
- Big soft brushes (for blush).
- Eyebrow brush.
- Tweezers.
- Blush.
- Eye shadows.
- Cover stick.
- Different lipsticks—all colors, including natural gloss.
- Mascara.
- Eyeliner.
- Nail polishes (3 or 4 different tints).
- Nail polish remover. (Pack nail polish and remover in leak-proof bag.)
- Little sponges (for foundation).
- Nail file or emery board.

- Brush and comb.
- Mirror.
- Hair accessories and curling iron, or hot rollers.

Obviously all these products and accessories must be in good condition, and you must renew them whenever necessary so that your kit is always complete. Certain articles of clothing are essential:

- Different panty hose.
- Lingerie (brassieres and panties), flesh color.

27

Helpful Information

Take time out before departure to learn the metric system, the twenty-four-hour clock, foreign clothing and shoe sizes, and other important terms. The more you can learn before you go the less traumatic the culture shock will be. This information is necessary for travel overseas.

Metric System

1 mile = 1.609 kilometers (km)

1 kilometer = 0.621 miles

1 yard = 0.914 meters (m)

1 meter = 1.094 yards

1 foot = 0.305 meters (m)

1 meter = 3.281 feet

1 inch = 2.54 centimeters (cm)

1 centimeter = 0.39 inches

1 pound = 0.453 kilograms (kg)

1 kilogram = 2.205 pounds

1 U.S. gallon = 3.785 liters (L)	1 liter = 0.264 U.S. gallons
1 imperial gallon = 4.545 liters	1 liter = 0.22 imperial gallons

Twenty-Four-Hour Clock

In the twenty-four-hour clock, each hour is referred to in hundreds, i.e. 1:00 A.M., is referred to as 0100 hours. As in the normal clock, the morning hours are 1–12; the afternoon hours are referred to as 1300 (thirteen hundred) hours to 2400 (twenty-four hundred) hours. Thus, 1:00 P.M. is 1300 hours. If you are given a time greater than 12:00 noon you have only to subtract 12 hundred in order to establish what that time would be, e.g. 1800 hours is 1800 – 1200 = 6:00 P.M. Practice this and you will find it easy to learn in either the standard or twenty-four-hour clock. The latter removes the ambiguity of A.M. and P.M.

Greenwich Mean Time (GMT)

You will hear this term in your travels. Greenwich (pronounced "Grennich") Mean Time is the standard time in Britain and the means by which standard time is measured around the world. Time in other countries is referred to as being behind (earlier than) GMT or ahead of (later than) GMT.

Temperature

To change Fahrenheit into centigrade subtract 32 from Fahrenheit and divide by 1.8. To convert centigrade into Fahrenheit, multiply centigrade by 1.8 and add 32.

International Telephone Direct Dialing

Direct dialing is not possible between all countries. To dial direct, you will need the international access code of the country you are in, plus the country code, plus the city code, plus the number. For example, to call Milan from the United States, you would dial 011 (international access code for the United States) plus 39 (country code for Italy) plus 2 (city code for Milan) plus number.

International Clothing Sizes

(Continental sizes are approximate)

WOMEN'S DRESSES

American	6	8	10
British	8	10	12
Continental	34/36	36/38	38/40
Australian	6	8	10

WOMEN'S SHOES

American	7	8	9
British	5½	6½	7½
Continental	38	40	41
Japanese	9.7	10.3	10.7

HOSIERY

American	8	8½	9	10
British	8	8½	9	10
Continental	0	1	2	4

MEN'S SUITS AND COATS

American	36	38	42
British	36	38	42
Continental	46	48	52
Australian	92	97	102

SHIRTS

American	14	14½	15	15½	16
British	14	14½	15	15½	16
Continental	36	37	38	39	41
Australian	36	37	38	39	40

MEN'S SHOES

American	8	8½	9	10	11
British	7½	8	8½	9½	10½
Continental	42	43	43	44	45

Models Mart

Models Mart, at 42 West 38th Street, Suite 802, New York, NY, 10018, is the international connection for models, actors, agents, and school directors. The authority here is David Vando, a playwright and actor, and the editor of the International Directory of Model and Talent Agencies and Schools, which is published by Peter Glenn Publications, Ltd. This directory is a worthwhile investment. David has been an advisor and friend to many people in the industry all over the world—including myself. In 1994, he was inducted into the Models Hall of Fame (the first inductee was the late, great Wilhelmina), which was founded by Betty Rasnic, another icon in the business, to honor those who have striven for excellence in serving the modeling profession. Here is David's advice for aspiring models: "Read, ask questions, and learn everything you can about the industry. The more you know, the better prepared you will be physically and mentally. You will be in a stronger position not to be taken advantage of by people who will trade on your aspirations. I would ask the models who are successful to make an effort to help those who would like to follow in their footsteps."

28

Competitions and Conventions

Model and talent competitions and conventions come and go. There is controversy over the value and validity of these events. Some are organized brilliantly and offer unquestionable value.

How can you evaluate a convention and how can you benefit from attending? Conventions afford young men and women the opportunity to discuss career potential and ambitions with experts in the industry. The purpose of these events is to bring together models and talent from all over the country, casting directors from Los Angeles and New York, and model agents from all over the world. Conventions vary in format but generally include competitions, workshops, seminars, callbacks, open interviews, and panel discussions. A well-run convention is beneficial to all concerned. Benefits include: contracts, trophies, advice from professionals, and deep insight into what is required in the modeling and acting professions. Parents have the opportunity to learn about the business. Agents and casting directors have a chance to scout for models and talent and to exchange ideas with colleagues.

If you plan to attend a convention, you must be assured that reputable agents will be present and that a specific time will be set aside for you to meet them. This is usually done during callbacks (the time allotted for agents to see models or talent in whom they have expressed a specific interest), or open interviews (another opportunity for all participants to see the agents of their choice). I must point out, however, that sometimes, at the last minute, a celebrity may become ill, a casting director may cancel because a casting has run much longer than expected or he or she has business requiring immediate attention, or a model agent may bow out because of sudden staff problems or the arrival of an out-of-town client. I have seen this happen on occasion. Unavoidable cancellations are understandable, but they can cause embarrassment and shake the credibility of the convention producer in the eyes of school directors, students, parents, and other agents. Be aware that this can happen and try to be understanding. By the same token convention planners would do well to drop an agent, casting director, or celebrity who makes a last-minute cancellation on two or more occasions.

A convention is not only a great opportunity to have fun, meet a lot of people, gain experience, and learn the business, it is also a launching pad for many careers. Models and actors are usually brought to these events by directors of modeling schools, promoters of model search events, or advertisements in the media. Some form of specialized preparation is advisable before participating in a convention. This can be obtained from most modeling schools.

Now let us discuss the financial aspect. There will be a registration fee and possible additional fees for competitions and workshops. Usually, the investment is worthwhile. You will meet the experts of the industry from all over the world, at one location, over the period of the convention (approximately 3–5 days). The alternative to attending a convention would involve traveling to New York, Chicago, Los Angeles, and foreign cities at great expense, without any guarantee that you would meet your chosen agency representatives. I can assure you that when convention planners are establishing fees, choosing hotels, and planning menus, the restricted budgets of the young people they hope to attract greatly influence their final decisions. I can also assure you that the cost of putting on a convention is great. The planning takes at least a year. Expenses include: travel and accommodation for agents and casting directors, lawyers' fees, a convention staff, security, a highly specialized technical crew, camera and video equipment, a stage production to showcase participating talent, and many other necessities.

I would suggest that you study the program of events well in advance with your school director. First-time participation at a convention can be an overwhelming experience. While the staff will be prepared to answer questions, the demands on their time are great. I have attended many conventions. A behind-the-scenes glimpse of my experiences will give you some idea of the problems the staff are expected to handle. There was the mother in the elevator who appeared to be having a heart attack but was in fact hyperventilating because her child did not win a competition! I remember the contestant who fell and, in true show business fashion, insisted on finishing her act. Later it was discovered she had broken her leg. In the same vein, there was the school director who was rushed to the hospital for an appendectomy only to return the next night complete with stitches, nurse, and doctor to see her school sweep to victory at an awards banquet. At the end of another convention I met one puzzled foreign agent who had missed the entire event by spending his stay at the wrong hotel—models are not the only people confused by a language barrier and a new location!

I asked some well-known personalities who have attended conventions for their views on these events. Mrs. Muriel Alt, who attended a convention with her daughter, top model Carol Alt, said: "I am amazed at the caliber of people who are here and at how accessible they are to the boys and girls.

At a convention like this young people can learn how much hard work is involved in the profession. They may also realize that acting and modeling is not for them. I feel only good can come out of this event." Carol told contestants: "You are very fortunate to have what this convention offers. Take advantage of the workshops. Get advice from the experts here."

Al Onorato (Onorato/Guillod), a respected personal manager, commented: "I think it provides an enormous link between people in the business and people who cannot just pick up and go to one of the major markets such as Los Angeles, New York, Chicago, or Europe. It gives me a chance to see untrained talent that may have some potential. It also gives me a chance to encourage them in that area or perhaps encourage them to explore other areas."

Allen Fawcett, coauthor of the book *Kid Biz,* said: "A convention is a means to an end. It is one step in a series of steps that must be taken in the pursuit of a career. It is about shopping your wares and about learning. If you are going to make mistakes, make them at a convention, not in the marketplace. If you have shortcomings, discover what they are before you go any further. Show business is a devastating profession for someone who has had a commodity called 'false hope' packaged and sold to them. A convention can be a valuable service if it is planned under controlled conditions."

Tony Shepherd, vice president of Aaron Spelling Productions, Los Angeles (Aaron Spelling has been responsible for more prime-time television than any other producer in the history of the media), was very enthusiastic. He said: "The competition is almost secondary to the benefits that the artists receive. These young people—I prefer to call them artists— have the opportunity to acquire a great deal of knowledge."

Helen Rogers and Pamela Edwards, her daughter, are the masterminds behind the International Modeling and Talent Association (IMTA) annual convention held in Los Angeles in January and in New York in July. This is a marathon of workshops, seminars, and competitions. Participants are brought to the convention by school directors, and both students and directors have access to the world's most notable casting directors and model agents. These experts judge contestants, discuss possible contracts during callbacks, and offer career guidance during open interviews.

School directors soak up information from panels, seminars, and workshops given by such experts as Nina Blanchard, Al Onorato, and Helen Rogers herself.

Helen, a former Ford model, told me: "After a modeling career in New York and Los Angeles, I opened a modeling school—Plaza 3 in Phoenix, Arizona. We made it as professional as it could possibly be. We had a tiny agency but we ran it like a New York agency. We had a very good reputation because we were honest.

"Plaza 3 became the largest-grossing school with the largest student enrollment in the country. We were accredited by the National Association of Trade and Technical Schools, and we introduced fashion merchandising, interior design, and commercial photography. Our modeling program was also accredited. Because of this accreditation we were able to obtain federal grant and loan programs. It also meant we had to have a placement office and a student guidance center.

"I was the most successful school director in the country and I made all the mistakes in the book. I don't want other school directors to make the same mistakes. I did lots of good things too. I want to share all of this with school owners and directors and encourage them to update their curriculum. As members of our organization they have the opportunity to have their students discovered by international agents. When an agent realizes that a school turns out good models, that school often becomes a recruitment source. There is no mystique about this. This is how it can and should work."

Pamela Edwards, senior vice president of IMTA, said: "This organization works because we are totally committed to making IMTA the best educational experience for the school directors and the talent. We are known internationally as the best discovery source for models and actors available anywhere. We listen to the input of everyone involved and implement suggestions wherever we can.''

The list of IMTA's successes is truly amazing. They include: Beverly Peele, Elija Wood, Ladd York, Joseph Beauchamp, and scores of film and television stars.

Here is what the experts say about IMTA conventions.

At an IMTA convention in Los Angeles, Nina Blanchard told school directors attending her seminar: ''I am very impressed with Helen Rogers. I know her ethics and that is why I am here. This is the only convention I have attended in fifteen years.''

Beatrice Traissac of International Beatrice Models in Milan was attending the same convention. She told me: ''I have been in the business for over twenty years and this is my first modeling convention. I respect Helen Rogers. She has a very serious convention. I've seen beautiful girls here and will be taking some back to Milan.''

The raves continue: Bill Arndt (BAMM, Los Angeles): ''IMTA is the highest caliber of talent presentation anywhere, and I happily signed some great guys.''

Paul Hagnauer (Best One Model Agency, Paris and Madrid): ''I have always found good models at this convention. Europe needs more and more new faces.''

Clair Sinnett (Clair Sinnett Casting, Bel Air, CA): ''It would take an actor years to meet the industry professionals he or she can meet in one week, under one roof, here at the IMTA convention. I wish I had had this opportunity when I was starting my career.''

Adam Hill (Adam Hill Actors Studio, Los Angeles): ''Integrity, talent, class, respect, and hard work permeate the entire convention.''

Judy La Grone (talent scout, New York/Los Angeles): ''IMTA is an unbeatable education for anyone who wants to be in this business.''

In conclusion, anyone who is interested in a modeling career and who has had little or no exposure to the business would be advised to attend a convention. I stated at the beginning of this chapter that competitions and conventions come and go. I advise you to check credentials before making any financial commitment. When you are satisfied, go to the convention, throw yourself into it, learn what you can, and enjoy a once-in-a-lifetime experience.

Here is a partial list of people who have had successful conventions, competitions, and model searches. They are listed in alphabetical order.

Facefinders World Class Model/Talent Expo. Contact: Tom and J. J. Meier, 3191 Tucker, Rossmoor, CA 90720. Tel. (714) 828-3223.

Ford Models Inc. "Supermodel of the World", 344 E. 59th Street, New York, NY 10022. Tel. (212) 735–6500.

International Model and Talent Association. Contact: Helen Rogers, P.O. Box 44726, Phoenix, AZ 85064. Tel. (602) 997-4907.

Millie Lewis American Model and Talent Competition, 510 Haddington Lane, Peach Tree City, GA 30269. Tel. (404) 487-6656.

"Look of the Year." Contact: Elite Models, 111 E. 22nd Street, New York, NY 10010. Tel. (212) 529-9700.

Modeling Association of America International. Contact: Betty Lane Gramling, 250 Doyle Street, Orangeburg, SC 29115. Tel. (803) 534-9672.

Modelling Association of Canada. Tel. (807) 345–2126.

Models of the South. Contact: R. Jack Rasnic, 907 Beveridge Road, Richmond, VA 23226. Tel. (804) 285-8450.

"New Faces" Model Search. Contact: Lucy Heim, 968 Pinetree Drive, Indian Harbour Beach, FL 32937. Tel. (407) 777-1344.

Wilhelmina Model Agency "Kid Search" (newborn to seventeen), 300 Park Avenue South, New York, NY 10010. Tel. (212) 473-0700.

This book is based on knowledge and advice from people who have been in the modeling business for many years. Sound basic principles and good advice never date.

Please remember that the only true failure is never having tried. Don't be afraid to try! What you can accomplish with the raw materials God has given you is up to you. Good luck with your career!